# AIR FRYER COOKBOOK

## *The Best Collection of Air Fryer Recipes For Your Home*

# Table of Contents

# Introduction

Sitting on your kitchen counter is one of the most popular appliances to date! Loved by both professional chefs and adventurous home cooks – like me, your air fryer is an easy to use and efficient appliance that you can just about cook anything in.

Now, if you haven't fallen in love with your air fryer yet my cookbook is just what you need! You'll see how easy it is to make amazing dishes with little to no grease including tender shrimp, kabobs and even s' mores. So, get ready to try these recipes for yourself with my handy cookbook filled with the best air fryer recipes for your home.

But before we get into creating your first meal, let's jump right into why your Air Fryer is such a big hit, the benefits of cooking with your air fryer and some awesome tips that will help you Air Fry like a pro!

## What's an Air Fryer?

Personally, I've never wondered about how my stove or fridge worked, and I bet you've haven't either. But with the air fryer it's a little bit different, right? Back when I first got my hands on my air fryer, I was so curious about how this appliance could fry foods with little to no oil. How is that even possible?

Now, I won't get too technical but here's what I found out. In short, your air fryer is basically a small turbo-powered convection oven. Yes, a convection oven! It works the same way by using a fast circulation of hot air to surround the food and cool it down quickly.

Your Air fryer does come equipped with a deep-fry basket, but there's no need to use a cup or more of oil.  The basket helps the heated air flow all around the food to bake it. So instead of oil-drenched food, you end up with fried food that is crispy on the outside and moist on the inside.

People also love the fact that it actually lives up to the hype, and delivers good and healthy food without a huge mess in the kitchen, which is a huge plus!

I'm sure you might have plenty of other questions you would like me to answer, so below I included a short Q&A of the most frequently asked questions.

### Do I have to preheat my air fryer?

Your air fryer heats up pretty fast so it all comes down to preference. You can either preheat it while you prep the ingredients or skip preheating and turn it on once the food is inside. Either way, you won't have to stand around waiting for your air fryer to get nice and hot like you would if you were cooking with an oven.

**Is air frying better than deep-frying?**

Yes, air frying is better than deep-frying! Instead of using cups of oil, you can easily fry chicken, French fries, and fish with a small amount of oil with your air fryer. You should also know that air fried food is more comparable to oven-fried foods, and not food that has been deep-fried. So instead of having that fatty fried flavor, your food will taste a lot leaner and healthier.

**Do I need to buy any extras and attachments for my air fryer?**

Most air fryers will include attachments such as pans and racks. These do come in handy when you want to cook breakfast dishes such as quiches and desserts like cakes. So, look into purchasing these extras;

***Flame Distributor:*** A flame distributor really comes in handy since it covers the food while it cooks in the air fryer. This accessory prevents oils and juices from splashing against the heating element, which is located right above the frying basket. It also prevents crumbs, nuts, and other small foods from flying up against the heating element.

***Grill Mat:*** A grill mat will keep the basket clean and allows for an easier clean-up. In addition, a grill mat can also be used just like the flame divider- preventing light foods or splashing of oils from touching the heating element. Keep in mind that the grill mat shouldn't touch the heating element either.

***Baking dish:*** For foods that are normally prepared in a casserole dish buy a baking dish that will fit into your air fryer. When you use a baking dish, just place it in the air fryer basket and then cook as usual.

**What can I cook in my air fryer?**

Just about anything can be cooked in your air fryer! Most people use it to cook meat, snacks, fries and much more. You can even make mini cakes, muffins, and cupcakes in the air fryer, or anything else you would like to bake.

When it comes to vegetables, you can air fry the same vegetables that you would put on the grill or in the oven. This includes corn, zucchini, potatoes, peppers, onion, and mushrooms, just to name a few. You can even make healthy kale chips and any other kinds veggie chips in your air fryer. A lot of people also turn to their air fryer to prepare frozen foods without defrosting them.

## How much can my air fryer hold?

Your standard air fryer can fit about 2 to 4 servings depending on the kind of food you're cooking. But no matter what, it's very important that you do not overcrowd the basket. If you do cook an air fryer recipe in multiple batches, check the second batch a few minutes early since the air fryer was already hot and this batch will cook more quickly.

## How do I prevent food from sticking to the inside of my air fryer?

I recommend spraying the basket lightly with vegetable oil spray or a light cooking spray when you what to cook foods that are prone to sticking, like breaded chicken or flakey fish. You can also use a foil sling which will make cleanup and the removal of certain foods easier, especially delicate fish.

## How do I clean my air fryer?

For starters, consult your air fryer manual before attempting to wash anything. The removable parts – the drawer and basket of many models, are dishwasher-safe. The main body of the air fryer should be wiped down occasionally since grease and food splatter can build up around the heat source and cause it to smoke. Just make sure your air fryer is completely cooled down before you touch the inside and use a mild detergent. After you clean the air fryer, run it briefly to dry the inside.

## What do I do if I smell smoke while air frying, or it smells funny?

Clean it! A smoky or a weird-smelling air fryer is normally caused by being dirty. So, if you smell something burning or see excessive smoke it's not your food burning, it's the residue around the heating element. Make sure you periodically clean any build-up residue around this important heating element.

Now that we're done with this helpful Q&A, we'll get into the full benefits to owning an Air Fryer and there's plenty!


## How Your Air Fryer Will Upgrade Your Life!

Thankfully, there are far more pros than cons with your amazing air fryer. For instance, your air fryer may not be able to cook every kind of food out there, but what it can cook it does so amazingly well! Below, I've listed seven awesome ways your Air Fryer will improve your lifestyle.

### 1. Better, Healthier Food

As we all know, deep-fried food isn't the healthiest for you and is connected to health problems such as heart disease and high cholesterol. When you cook with your air fryer it helps to cut down on the amount of oil you use to cook each meal while giving you the flavors you love. All you need is a small amount of oil to get similar results!  Plus, you can easily chop up veggies such as zucchinis, sweet potatoes, and Brussel sprouts to enjoy in no time and get your daily recommended serving of vegetables.

## 2. A Small Space Saver

Whether you have a small kitchen or you're living in a shared space like a dorm room, your small air fryer is an amazing appliance to own. It's roughly the size of a coffee maker, yet cooks like a traditional convection oven and can be stored away when it's not in use.

## 3. Faster Cook Times

Your air fryer works so well since it's so small and powerful! When compared to an oven, on average it can take up to 10-15 minutes to simply preheat. Your air fryer, on the other hand, heats up and is ready to use in minutes.  For example, cooking frozen fries would take a good 45 minutes in the oven, but in an air fryer you can be eating them in just 15. That's a 30-minute difference! So, when you're in need of a quick snack or meal, without a doubt it's best to use your air fryer.

## 4. All-In-One Cooking Style

Sure, your air fryer can cook French fries really well, but it can do so much more! Get ready to bake, grill, broil, roast and even stir fry meats and vegetables. You can also cook fresh and frozen foods when you're short on time, and use your air fryer to reheat leftovers.

Trust me, you'll love keeping your stove off and cooking everything from fresh fish, sweets, toasted sandwiches, and fresh vegetables in your Air Fryer.  If you go shopping for more attachments and accessories like a roasting rack and grill pan, you'll be able to do even more!

## 5. Easy Clean-Up

Love cooking, but hate the messy clean-up? Then you'll love using your air fryer! The best part of about this appliance is the fact that you can quickly clean the basket and inner pan thanks to they're non-stick surfaces. Instead of taking hours of soaking to clean up after a meal or snack it will take minutes.

## 6. Super Easy to Use

No confusing instructions here! Your air fryer has an easy to follow interface that anyone can use. Just select the correct temperature for your food and add the cooking time, place the food inside, and don't forget to give it a few shakes while it cooks. Also, there's no need to preheat the air fryer or continuously watch over it like you would with a pan on the stove.

Also, the baskets make shaking your food simple and fast too. So, you can check and shake your food without decreasing the internal heat and slowing down the cooking process.

## 7. Energy Efficiency

It's always good to have energy-efficient appliances like your air fryer since it will save you money in the long run. The air fryer also produces zero extra heat you won't have to cool down your house when you cook with it in the summertime, which means bonus savings for you!

# Do's & Don't to Air Fry Like A Pro

Want to cook like an air frying pro? Skip all those beginner mistakes and use your air fryer to its full potential with the following Do's and Don'ts!

## DO Cook with Oven base recipes

Good news! You can use an oven recipe in your air fryer and not miss out on all those great recipes. So, when you come across a tasty recipe for amazing oven-baked chicken or seasoned steak that's made for a conventional oven don't skip over it, just adjust the recipe to suit your air fryer.

You can do this by lowering the cooking temperature by about 25°F and subtract 20% of the original cooking time – although this can vary on what you choose to cook. Once you're done, you'll have a new air fryer recipe to try!

## DO bake in your air fryer

Baking just got a whole lot easier thanks to your air fryer! Enjoy breads, cinnamon rolls, and small cakes that are made in minutes rather than hours because of your air fryer's super-fast airflow. Just purchase a few small pans and bundt pans, and you're all set to create some amazing desserts.

## DON'T overload the basket

Filling your basket all the way up with food like you would a traditional deep-fryer is just a bad idea. You can cause the food to that is either burn or not cook properly. This happens because the air fryer doesn't use cups of oil, it simply cooks your food with hot air from every angle. So, if you don't remember to work in batches, you'll be left with a meal you can't eat.

You also what to make sure that there is plenty of space around your food and you shake it halfway through cooking for evenly crispy results.

## DO air-fry more veggies

Vegetables are awesome when cooked in your air fryer! Try roasting a few of your favorite vegetables and you'll definitely be blown away with how they turn out. Chop them up or leave them whole, air fryer and then enjoy vegetables are tender in the inside and caramelized, and a bit crunchy on the outside.

## DON'T use a wet batter

Fry as many foods as you want in your air fryer, just don't use a wet batter or coating on your food. Unfortunately, your air fryer can't make the batter crispy on the outside the way hot oil does. So instead of having a nice crispy shell, you'll end up with a dripping wet batter mess. You can get the crunch you want without the mess by opting to dredge your food in flour, beaten eggs, and breadcrumbs or panko.

## DO Shake Things Up

Plan on cooking fried food like nuggets, veggies, chicken nuggets, etc you have to shake your air fryer occasionally to get things cooking right. When you move things around halfway through the cooking process you help to make sure that the air surrounds food and cooks evenly for crispy results.

## DO add a splash of oil before cooking

Yes, you can get away with cooking crispy foods with zero oil in your air fryer. But with just a little bit of oil sprinkle on before cooking, you can change up the color, texture, and taste of the dish. Remember, oil has fat in it that helps to brown and season your food. So, before you place your food in the air fryer spray it with a non-stick cooking spray or light sprinkle of olive oil.

## DON'T spray nonstick spray directly into the Air Fryer cooking the basket

Like I mentioned above, you need to spray the food. But please DO NOT spray the actual cooking basket with nonstick spray since the chemicals found in it can actually work against the already nonstick basket. Just simply spray the food on a rack or plate before placing it into the basket.

Or you can skip the commercial aerosol sprays and DIY-it with natural oils. Just purchase a hand-pump oil sprayer and fill it with heart-friendly oil — olive, avocado, etc — and spray your food or spritz the basket.

## DO use your air fryer more than your microwave

Microwaved leftovers are notorious for tasting different from the night before. They're usually less crispy and rubbery. On the other hand, your air fryer will reheat and re-crisp your food perfectly! You can also reheat frozen package foods in your air fryer too.

**DON'T cook foods that require liquids.**

You can definitely crisp up dishes that are made with rice, pasta and other grains in your air fryer with a little oil, but you shouldn't actually try to cook them in the air fryer. Your air fryer can't boil water so it's best to cook them as directed.

# Recipe Introduction

Now that you know more about how your Air Fryer works, the lifestyle benefits of having one and plenty of pro tips, it's time to start cooking! My cookbook is full of the best Air Fry recipes that are easy to create and most importantly delicious. Whether you're an on-the-go mom, busy college student or a home cook looking to save some time, you'll have no problem creating an amazing dish for breakfast, lunch, and dinner with my Air Fryer Cookbook.

# Breakfast

## *Classic French Toast*

*Topped with powdered sugar and whipped cream, these French toast recipe is a  sweet treat in the morning!*

Prep Time: 5 Minutes

Cook Time: 6 Minutes

Total Time: 11 Minutes

Servings: 1

## Ingredients:

- 4 pieces bread, of your choice and desired thickness
- 2 Tbsp butter or margarine, softened
- 2 eggs, gently beaten
- 1 pinch cinnamon
- 1 pinch nutmeg
- 1 pinch ground cloves
- 1 pinch salt
- 1 tsp icing sugar and/or maple syrup for garnish and serving

## Directions:

1. Preheat the air fryer to 350 degrees F
2. In a bowl, add in the two eggs, gently beat together, add in a sprinkle of salt, a few heavy shakes of cinnamon, and small pinches of ground nutmeg and ground cloves
3. Butter each side of the bread slices, cut into strips
4. Dredge each strip in the egg mixture and arrange in air fryer (you will be working in two batches).
5. After 2 minutes of cooking, pause the air fryer, remove the pan, and place on a heat safe surface, then spray the bread with cooking spray
6. Once the strips are generously, flip and spray the second side as well
7. Return pan to fryer, cook for 4 more minutes, making sure to check on it after a couple minutes to ensure they are cooking evenly
8. Once the eggs are cooked and the bread is a golden brown, remove from air fryer and serve immediately
9. Serve with a sprinkle icing sugar, whip cream, drizzle with maple syrup, or serve with syrup for dipping.

**Nutrition Facts** Per Serving: Calories:178 |Protein: 5g |Total Fat: 15g|Total Carbs: 2g

## *Loaded Veggie Omelet*

*Customize your own fluffy omelet by loading it up with fresh veggies and meats of your choice, and air frying it for less than 8 minutes!*

Prep Time: 5 Minutes

Cook Time: 8 Minutes

Total Time: 13 Minutes

Servings: 1

## Ingredients:

- 2 eggs
- 1/4 cup milk
- Pinch of salt
- Fresh meat and veggies of your choice, diced (red bell pepper, green onions, ham and mushrooms)
- 1 tsp Breakfast Seasoning of your choice
- 1/4 cup shredded cheddar and mozzarella cheese

## Directions:

1. Preheat the air fryer to 350 degrees F
2. In a small bowl, mix together the eggs and milk, stir well to combined, then add in a pinch of salt
3. In a bowl, add in the veggies and meat of your choice
4. Pour the egg mixture into a well-greased 6"x3" pan, making sure to pour carefully
5. Place the pan into the basket of the air fryer
6. Air fry for 8-10 minutes
7. Once halfway cooked through, sprinkle the eggs with the breakfast seasoning of your choice and top with the cheese
8. Once cooked, remove the pan and with a thin spatula, loosen the omelet from the sides of the pan and transfer to a plate
9. Top with extra green onions and enjoy!

**Nutrition Facts** Per Serving: Calories:244 |Protein: 23g |Total Fat: 11g|Total Carbs: 14g

### ***Toasted Coconut French Toast***

*Made with just 4 ingredients, this classic French toast recipe has a fun tropical twist. Serve it with pineapple jam to complete the tropical taste.*

Prep Time: 10 Minutes

Cook Time: 4 Minutes

Total Time: 14 Minutes

Servings: 1

**Ingredients:**

- 2 slices of semi-thick bread, your choice
- 1/2 cup coconut milk
- 1 tsp baking powder
- 1/2 Cup Unsweetened Shredded Coconut

**Directions:**

1. In a bowl, combine the coconut milk and baking powder
2. On a plate, spread the shredded coconut
3. Take each slice of bread, first soak in the coconut milk mixture and a few seconds before transferring to the plate with the shredded coconut and fully coating the slice in the coconut
4. Make sure there is space between the coated slices of bread in the air fryer, close it, and set the temperature to 350 degrees F and cook 4 minutes
5. Once done, remove and enjoy with pineapple jam or maple syrup or your favorite French toast toppings!

**Nutrition Facts** Per Serving: Calories:558 |Protein: 7g |Total Fat: 42g|Total Carbs: 44g

### *Crispy Bacon*

*Forget all the popping grease or splatter, enjoy perfect crispy bacon in just 10 minutes with zero fuss!*

Prep Time: 1 Minutes

Cook Time: 9 Minutes

Total Time: 10 Minutes

Servings: 2

**Ingredients:**

- 3-7 Pieces Bacon

**Directions:**

1. At the bottom of the air fryer, arrange a single layer of bacon
2. Air Fry the bacon at 350 degrees F for 9 minutes (thick cut bacon) or shorter for thinner bacon – making sure to check on the bacon while it cooks so it doesn't overcook
3. Transfer the cook to a plate
4. Enjoy with scrambled eggs and pancakes or in a breakfast sandwich

**Recipe Notes:** After the air fryer has cooled, take a damp cloth and wipe any grease that has splattered.

**Nutrition Facts** Per Serving: Calories:256 |Protein: 8g |Total Fat: 26g|Total Carbs: 1g

### ***Donuts & Holes***

*Now you can grab a donut or a few holes for breakfast thanks to this oh so easy recipe anyone can create!*

Prep Time: 1 Minutes

Cook Time: 9 Minutes

Total Time: 10 Minutes

Yields 8 donuts and 8 holes

## Ingredients:

- 1 can layered biscuits
- 3 tbsp melted butter
- 1/3 cup granulated sugar
- 1/2 to 1 tsp cinnamon (adjust to your taste)
- 4 tbsp dark brown sugar, clumps broken up
- Pinch of allspice

## Directions:

1. In a bowl, combine the sugar, cinnamon, brown sugar, and allspice in a small, and set aside
2. Remove biscuits from can (do not flatten), use a 1-inch circle biscuit cutter to cut the holes out of the center of each biscuit
3. Arrange the Donuts in the Air Fryer and air fry at 350 F for 5 minutes, working in batches of 4 donuts
4. Then Air fry the Holes at 350 F for 3 minutes, working in batches of 8 holes
5. As each batch of donuts and holes is cooked and removed from the fryer, use a pastry brush to top the entire surface of each donut and hole with butter
6. After each donut and hole are topped with butter, dunk into the bowl with the sugar mixture and coat completely with the mixture, then gently shake off excess
7. Enjoy!

**Nutrition Facts** Per Serving of 2: Calories:151 |Protein: .66g |Total Fat: 9g|Total Carbs: 16g

### *Hard "Boiled" Eggs*

*Just add the eggs, no water needed!*

Prep Time: 1 Minutes

Cook Time: 15-17 Minutes

Total Time: 16-18 Minutes

Servings: 2-4

**Ingredients:**

- 4 large eggs
- Salt, black pepper
- Everything bagel seasoning, optional

**Directions:**

1. Place all the eggs in the air fryer basket
2. Cook at 250F for 15 minutes for a softer yolk, or 17 minutes for a firmer yolk (time will vary depending on the make and model of your air fryer)
3. Remove the eggs, under cold water and peel right away
4. Enjoy with toast or alone seasoned with salt, black pepper or everything bagel seasoning

**Nutrition Facts** Per Serving: Calories:55 |Protein: 2g |Total Fat: 4g|Total Carbs: 0.65g

# *Blueberry and Lemon Muffin*

*Blueberries and lemons, such a beautiful combination! Create these yummy muffins in no time with this recipe that is perfect for breakfast or brunch!*

Prep Time: 5-8 Minutes

Cook Time: 10 –12 Minutes

Total Time: 25-35 Minutes

Yields: 1 dozen

## Ingredients:

- 2 1/2 cups self-rising flour
- 1/2 cup Monk Fruit or sweetener of your choice
- 1/2 cup cream
- 1/4 cup avocado oil or any light cooking oil
- 2 eggs
- 1 cup blueberries
- Zest from 1 lemon
- Juice from 1 lemon
- 1 tsp vanilla
- Brown sugar, to sprinkle on top

## Directions:

1. In small bowl, mix together the self-rising flour and sugar, set aside
2. In a medium bowl, combine the cream, oil, lemon juice, eggs and vanilla
3. Add the flour mixture to the wet mixture and stir just until blended, then stir in the blueberries
4. Spoon the batter into single silicone cupcake holders, then sprinkle ½ tsp brown sugar on top of each muffin
5. Preheat the Air fryer to 320 degrees F
6. Air Fry the muffins for 10 minutes, check the muffins at 6 minutes to make sure that they are not cooking too fast – Check the muffins by placing a toothpick into the center of the muffin, if the toothpick comes out clean and the muffins are lightly brown, they are done.
7. Once done, remove the muffins and allow them to cool
8. Enjoy!

**Recipe Notes:** No need to over-bake the muffins, they'll cook for another minute or so after they are transferred to a plate.

**Nutrition Facts** Per Muffin: Calories:198 |Protein: 4g |Total Fat: 7g|Total Carbs: 29g |

## *Tofu and Broccoli Scramble*

*Not in the mood for eggs? Then try this healthy alternative scramble made with tofu, broccoli and potato all seasoned to perfection!*

Prep Time: 10 Minutes

Cook Time: 40 Minutes

Total Time: 50 Minutes

Servings: 4

## Ingredients:

- 1 block tofu - chopped into 1" pieces
- 4 cups broccoli florets
- 2 1/2 cups chopped red potato - 1" cubes, 2-3 potatoes
- 1/2 cup chopped onion
- 2 tbsp soy sauce
- 1 tbsp olive oil
- 1 tsp turmeric
- 1/2 tsp garlic powder
- 1/2 tsp onion powder
- 1 tbsp olive oil

## Directions:

1. In a medium sized bowl, toss the tofu with the soy sauce, olive oil, turmeric, garlic powder, onion powder, and onion, set aside to marinate
2. In a separate bowl, toss the potatoes in the olive oil, and air fry at 400F for 15 minutes, shaking after 7-8 minutes into cooking
3. Shake the potatoes again, then add in the tofu, reserving any leftover marinade
4. Set the tofu and potatoes to cook at 370F for 15 more minutes, and start the air fryer
5. While the tofu is cooking, toss and cover the broccoli in the reserved marinade - If there isn't enough to cover the broccoli, add in a little extra soy sauce
6. When there are 5 minutes of cooking time remaining, add the broccoli to the air fryer
7. Once done, transfer to the tofu scramble to a plate
8. Enjoy!

**Nutrition Facts** Per Serving: Calories:272 |Protein: 7g |Total Fat: 9g |Total Carbs: 42g

# ***Cinnamon Rolls***

*Cinnamon rolls are the best! Enjoy this air fryer version that cooks in just 5 minutes with this easy and tasty recipe.*

Prep Time: 1 hr 30 Minutes

Cook Time: 5 Minutes

Total Time: 1 hr 35 Minutes

Servings: 8

## Ingredients:

- 1 lb frozen bread dough, thawed
- ¼ cup butter, melted and cooled
- 1½ tbsp ground cinnamon
- ¾ cup brown sugar

*Cream Cheese Glaze:*

- 2 tbsp butter, softened
- 1¼ cups powdered sugar
- 4 oz cream cheese, softened
- ½ tsp vanilla

## Directions:

1. Place the bread dough on a flat surface and allow to reach room temperature
2. Lightly floured the surface, roll the dough into a 13-inch by 11-inch rectangle and then position the rectangle on the 13-inch side facing you
3. Brush the melted butter over the dough, all while keeping a 1-inch border uncovered on the edge farthest away from you
4. In a bowl, combine the cinnamon and brown sugar
5. Sprinkle the mixture evenly over the buttered dough – keeping the 1-inch border uncovered
6. Roll the dough into the shape of a log starting with the edge closest to you, continue to roll the dough tightly - making sure to evenly roll and push out any air pockets. When you reach the uncovered edge of dough, press the dough onto the roll to seal everything together.
7. Divide the log into 8 pieces by slicing the log slowly with a sawing motion to make sure you don't flatten the dough, then turn the slices on their sides and cover with a clean kitchen towel, allow the rolls to sit and rise in the warmest part of the kitchen for 1½ to 2 hours
8. Prepare the glaze by placing the butter and cream cheese and butter – To soften the mixture, microwave for 30 seconds at a time until it is easy to stir. Then gradually add in the powdered sugar and stir to combine. Next, add in the vanilla extract and whisk until smooth, set aside

9.  Once the rolls have risen, pre-heat the air fryer to 350 degrees F, then transfer 4 of the rolls to the air fryer basket and air-fry for 5 minutes, then turn the rolls over and air-fry for another 4 minutes. Repeat this set with the remaining 4 rolls.
10. Allow the rolls to cool for a couple of minutes before glazing them with the cream cheese glaze
11. Serve warm and enjoy!

**Nutrition Facts** Per Serving: Calories:431 |Protein: 6g |Total Fat: 18g|Total Carbs: 64g

## Biscuit Pockets

*Fluffy and flakey, these amazing little sandwiches are filled with egg, sausage, and cheese, and ready to devour in 45 minutes!*

Prep Time: 30 Minutes

Cook Time: 15 Minutes

Total Time: 45 Minutes

Servings: 10

### Ingredients:

- 1 can (10.2 oz) Pillsbury grands!  Flaky Layers refrigerated biscuits (5 biscuits)
- 2 oz sharp cheddar cheese, cut in ten 1/2-inch cubes
- ¼ lb bulk breakfast sausage
- 1 tbsp vegetable oil
- 2 eggs, beaten
- 1/8 tsp salt
- 1/8 tsp pepper

*Egg Wash:*

- 1 egg
- 1 tbsp water

### Directions:

1. Cut two 8-inch rounds of cooking parchment paper, place one round in the bottom of air fryer basket, then spray with cooking spray
2. In 10-inch nonstick skillet over medium-high heat, add the oil
3. Once heated, add the sausage and cook for 2-5 minutes, stirring occasionally to crumble and until no longer pink, using slotted spoon, transfer to medium bowl. Then reduce the heat to medium, then add in the beaten eggs, salt and pepper to drippings in skillet, cook until eggs are thickened but still moist, stirring frequently. Place the eggs and sausage into bowl, stir and allow to cool for 5 minutes
4. In the meantime, separate dough into 5 biscuits and separate each biscuit into 2 layers - press each into a 4-inch round pan
5. Spoon 1 heaping tbsp of the egg and sausage mixture egg mixture onto the center of each round, then top with one piece of the cheese. Gently fold the edges up and over filling, pinch to seal
6. In a small bowl, beat the remaining egg and water together, brush the biscuits on all sides with egg wash.
7. Place 5 of the biscuit pockets, seam sides down, on parchment in air fryer basket, spray both sides of second parchment round with the cooking spray
8. Top the biscuit pockets in the basket with second parchment round, then top with remaining 5 biscuit pockets
9. Set the Air Fryer to 325 degrees F cook 8 minutes

10. Remove the top parchment round, using tongs, carefully turn biscuits, and place in basket in single layer Cook for 4-6 minutes longer or until cooked through

**Recipe Note:** If anything, don't skip the parchment paper! You need to separate these pockets or they will stick together.

**Nutrition Facts** Per Serving: Calories:176 |Protein: 7g |Total Fat: 10g |Total Carbs: 15g

### *Veggie Frittata*

*Loaded with healthy mushrooms, tomatoes, and fresh chives, this veggie frittata is perfect for breakfast!*

Prep Time: 5 Minutes

Cook Time: 15 Minutes

Total Time: 20 Minutes

Servings: 1

**Ingredients:**

- 1 cup egg whites
- 2 tbsp skim milk
- ¼ cup sliced tomatoes
- ¼ cup sliced mushrooms
- 2 tbsp chopped fresh chives
- Black pepper, to taste
- Salt, to taste

**Directions:**

1. Preheat Air Fryer at 320 degrees F
2. In a bowl, whisk together the egg whites, sliced tomatoes, mushrooms, chopped chives, salt and pepper
3. Pour the egg mixture to a greased circular pan or to the bottom of the air fryer after removing the accessory
4. Air Fryer for 15 minutes or until frittata is cooked through
5. Gently remove the frittata
6. Enjoy!

**Nutrition Facts** Per Serving: Calories:148 |Protein: 28g |Total Fat: 1g |Total Carbs: 4g

## Homemade Strawberry Pop Tarts

*Kids and adults will love these healthier homemade Strawberry Pop Tarts! They're so easy to make and taste amazing.*

Prep Time: 15 minutes

Cook Time: 10 minutes

Total Time: 25 minutes

Servings 6

### Ingredients:

- 2 refrigerated pie crusts
- 1 tsp cornstarch
- 1 tsp sugar sprinkles
- 1 tsp stevia
- 1/3 cup low-sugar strawberry preserves, organic
- 1/2 cup plain, non-fat vanilla Greek yogurt
- 1 oz reduced-fat Philadelphia cream cheese
- Olive oil or coconut oil spray

### Directions:

1. On a flat working surface, lay out the pie crust
2. Using a knife or pizza cutter, cut the 2 pie crusts into 6 rectangles (3 from each pie crust), each needs to be fairly long in length to fold it over and close the pop tart
3. In a bowl, add the preserves and cornstarch, stir and mix well
4. Add in a tbsp of the preserve mixture to the crust, place the preserves in the upper area of the crust
5. Fold each over to close the pop tarts, then use a fork to make imprints in each of the pop tarts to create vertical and horizontal lines along the edges.
6. Place the pop tarts in the Air Fryer and spray with oil
7. Cook on 375 degrees for 10 minutes, checking after 8 minutes to make sure they are not too crispy
8. In a bowl, combine the Greek yogurt, cream cheese, and stevia in a bowl to create the frosting
9. Allow the Pop Tarts to cool before removing them from the Air Fryer or they may break
10. Once cooled, remove the pop tarts from the Air Fryer
11. Top each one with the frosting and sprinkle with the sugar sprinkles

**Recipe Notes:** Cook only 2-3 Pop Tarts at a time.  You can stack them and then pull them apart once they have cooled.

**Nutrition Facts** Per Serving: Calories:322 |Protein: 4g |Total Fat: 18g |Total Carbs: 34g

## *Puffed Egg Tarts*

*Flakey with a yummy egg middle, these Puffed Eggs Tarts are just what you want for breakfast!*

Prep Time: 10 Minutes

Cook Time: 40 Minutes

Total Time: 50 Minutes

Servings: 4

## Ingredients:

- 4 large eggs
- 1 sheet frozen puff pastry half a 17.3-oz, thawed
- All-purpose flour, to dust
- 3/4 cup shredded cheese such as Gruyère, Cheddar or Monterey Jack, divided
- 1 tbsp minced fresh parsley or chives, optional

## Directions:

1. Preheat air fryer to 390 degrees F
2. On a lightly floured surface, unfold the thawed pastry sheet, then cut into 4 squares
3. Place 1 squares in air fryer basket, air-fry for 10 minutes or until pastry is light golden brown
4. Open basket and then using a metal spoon to press down the centers of each square in order to make an indentation
5. Sprinkle each indentation with 3 tbsp of cheese and carefully crack an egg into the center of each pastry, continue to air-fry for 7-11 minutes or until eggs are cooked to your desired doneness
6. Using oven pads, carefully transfer the puffed egg tarts to a wire rack set over waxed paper, allow to cool for 5 minutes
7. Repeat steps 3 to 7 with the remaining pastry squares, cheese, and eggs
8. If desired, sprinkle with half the parsley
9. Serve warm and enjoy!

**Recipe Notes**: Always use mitts when touching the basket. Also, before adding the egg to the pastry, crack the egg in a cup and pour into the puff pastry.

**Nutrition Facts** Per Serving: Calories:189 |Protein: 9g |Total Fat: 15g |Total Carbs: 5g

### ***Breakfast Baked Apple***

*Nothing like a delicious baked apple to start your day with! Got pears on hand? You can use them too!*

Prep Time: 5 Minutes

Cook Time: 20 Minutes

Total Time: 25 Minutes

Servings: 1

## Ingredients:

- 1 medium apple or pear
- 1 ½ tsp light margarine or butter, melted
- ¼ tsp cinnamon
- ¼ tsp nutmeg
- 2 tbsp chopped walnuts
- 2 tbsp raisins
- ¼ cup water

## Directions:

1. Preheat air fryer to 350 degrees F
2. Prepare the apples or pear by splitting them in half around the middle and spoon out some of the flesh.
3. Place the apple or pear in frying pan accessory or at the bottom of the air fryer after removing the accessory
4. In a small bowl, combine the margarine, cinnamon, nutmeg, walnuts and raisins
5. Spoon this mixture into the centers of the apple or pear halves.
6. Pour water into the pan
7. Air fry for 20 minutes or until the apples or pears have browned
8. Allow to cool and enjoy!

**Nutrition Facts** Per Serving: Calories:251 |Protein: 4g |Total Fat: 15g |Total Carbs: 28g

## *Hash Browns*

*This hash brown recipe is just what you need when you're in a hurry! Eat them alone or served them up with eggs, sausage and fresh fruit for a complete breakfast.*

Prep Time: 15 Minutes

Cook Time: 15 Minutes

Total Time: 30 Minutes

Servings: 3-4

## Ingredients:

- 4 Large potatoes, peeled and finely grated
- 2 tbsp, corn flour
- 2 tsp chili flakes, or to taste
- 1 tsp garlic powder
- 1 tsp onion powder, optional
- 1 + 1 tsp vegetable oil
- Salt, to taste
- Pepper powder, to taste

## Directions:

1. In a large bowl, soak the shredded potatoes in cold water, drain the water and repeat the step to drain excess starch from potatoes
2. In a non-stick pan, heat 1 tsp of vegetable oil and sauté shredded potatoes till cooked slightly for 3-4 minutes
3. Allow the potatoes to cool down and transfer the potatoes to a plate
4. Add the corn flour, salt, pepper, garlic and onion powder and chili flakes, mix together roughly
5. Spread over the plate and pat it firmly with your fingers.
6. Refrigerate the potatoes for 20 minutes
7. Preheat the Air Fryer to 350 degrees F
8. Remove the refrigerated potato and divide into equal pieces with a knife
9. Brush the wire basket of the air fryer with a little bit of oil
10. Place the hash brown pieces in the basket and air fry for 15 minutes at 350 degrees F
11. After 6 minutes, take the out the basket and flip the hash browns, then continue to cook
12. Serve hot with ketchup

**Nutrition Facts** Per Serving: Calories:320 |Protein: 8g |Total Fat: 2g |Total Carbs: 70g

## *Perfect Sausages*

*Have sausage in the freezer? Forget about cooking it on the oven, place it in the air fryer and serve it up with red and green sliced peppers or your breakfast food favorites.*

Cook Time:20 minutes

Total Time:20 minutes

Servings: 5

**Ingredients:**

- 5 raw and uncooked sausage links, of your choice

**Directions:**

- Prepare the air fryer by lining the basket with parchment paper, this will soak up grease and prevent it from smoking
- Place the sausage on top of the paper, it's okay if they touch
- Cook for 15 minutes on 360 F, open and then flip, continue to cook for an additional 5 minutes or until the sausage reaches an internal temperature of 160 F
- Allow the sausage to cool before serving with your favorite breakfast foods

**Nutrition Facts** Per Serving: *depends on your brand of sausage*

## *Cheesy Vegetable Quiche*

*Dig into this amazing cheesy vegetable quiche for breakfast! The fluffy eggs are loaded with healthy veggies and topped with cheese.*

Prep Time: 10 Minutes

Cook Time: 40 Minutes

Total Time: 50 Minutes

Servings: 2

### Ingredients:

- 3 large carrots, diced
- 1 large tomato, chopped
- 1 large broccoli, florets, chopped
- 7 tbsp cheddar cheese, grated
- 1 tbsp feta cheese
- 150 ml whole milk
- 2 large eggs, beaten
- 1 tsp parsley
- 1 tsp thyme
- Salt, to taste
- Pepper, to taste

### Directions:

1. Prepare the vegetables by chopping up the broccoli into florets, then peel and dice the carrots, place the carrots and broccoli into a food steamer and cook for 20 minutes or until soft
2. In a measuring cup add the seasonings (parsley, thyme, salt and pepper), crack the eggs into the cup and mix well, add in the milk a little at a time until the mixture is pale
3. Once the steamer is done, drain the vegetables and spread on the bottom of the quiche dish, layer with the tomatoes and top with cheese
4. Pour the liquid over and then add a little more cheese on top
5. Place in the air fryer, cook for 20 minutes on 350F
6. Once the quiche is cooked through, top with the feta and serve!

**Recipe Note:** If you don't think you can crack your eggs directly into the measuring cup, then crack them in a bowl first and then add them to the measuring cup.

**Nutrition Facts** Per Serving: Calories:488 |Protein: 31g |Total Fat: 26g |Total Carbs: 36g

# *Cranberry Pecan Muffins*

*Enjoy a delicious cranberry pecan muffin in the morning with your favorite hot or cold drink!*

Prep Time: 10 Minutes or less

Cook Time: 15 Minutes

Total Time: 25-35 Minutes

Yields: 6-8 muffins

## Ingredients:

- 1/4 cup cashew milk or use any dairy or non-dairy milk you prefer
- 2 large eggs
- 1/4 cup chopped pecans
- 1/2 cup fresh cranberries
- 1/2 tsp vanilla extract
- 1 1/2 cups Almond Flour
- 1/4 cup Monkfruit or a preferred sweetener
- 1 tsp baking powder
- 1/4 tsp cinnamon
- 1/8 tsp salt
- White chocolate, if desired

## Directions:

1. In a blender jar, add the milk, eggs and vanilla extract and blend 20-30 seconds, then add in the baking powder, almond flour, sugar, cinnamon and salt, blend another 30-45 seconds until well combined
2. Removed the blender jar from the base and stir in the 1/2 of the pecans and fresh cranberries
3. Pour the mixture to silicone muffin cups, top all of the muffins with the rest of fresh cranberries
4. Place the muffins into the air fryer basket and bake on 325 degrees F for 12 to 15 minutes or until the toothpick comes out clean
5. Remove from air fryer and allow to cool on wire rack
6. Drizzle with a maple glaze and a drizzled melted white chocolate, if desired

**Nutrition Facts** Per Serving: Calories:108 |Protein: 1g |Total Fat: 5g |Total Carbs: 13g

### ***Breakfast Bacon Grilled Cheese***

*Fix an amazing breakfast sandwich in just a few minutes with this bacon grilled cheese recipe! Serve it up with fresh fruit for a complete breakfast.*

Prep Time: 5 minutes

Cook Time: 7 minutes

Total Time: 12 minutes

Servings 2

## Ingredients:

- 4 slices of bread
- 1 tbsp butter melted
- 2 slices mozzarella cheese
- 2 slices mild cheddar cheese
- 5-6 slices cooked bacon

## Directions:

1. Add the butter to a bowl, heat in the microwave for 10-15 seconds to soften
2. Spread the butter onto one side of each of the slices of bread
3. Take one slice of bread and place it butter side down onto the air fryer basket
4. Top with the remaining ingredients in the following order: slice of cheddar cheese, sliced cooked bacon, and a slice of mozzarella cheese, then top with another slice of bread butter side up
5. If need, use a layer rack or trivet to hold down the sandwich to keep it from flying around inside the air fryer
6. Cook for 4 minutes on 370 degrees F
7. Open the air fryer, flip the sandwich and cook for an additional 3 minutes
8. Remove the sandwich and serve!

**Recipe Notes:** Depending on the size of your air fryer you can cook more than one sandwich, stacking sandwiches is not recommended.

**Nutrition Facts** Per Serving: Calories:642 |Protein: 27g |Total Fat: 49g |Total Carbs: 21g

# *Apple Cinnamon Empanadas*

*Enjoy these Air Fryer Apple Cinnamon Empanadas in just 20 minutes or make ahead for an easy grab and go breakfast.*

Prep Time: 15 Minutes

Cook Time: 18 Minutes

Total Time: 33 Minutes

Servings: 12

## Ingredients:

- 2 apples diced, 1 one red and 1 green
- 12 empanada wrappers
- 2 tbsp raw honey
- 1 tsp vanilla extract
- 1 tsp cinnamon
- 1/8 tsp nutmeg
- 1 tsp olive oil spray
- 2 tsp cornstarch
- 1 tsp water

## Directions:

1. In a saucepan over medium-high heat, add the apples, cinnamon, nutmeg, honey, and vanilla, stir and cook for 2-3 minutes or until the apples have soften
2. In a small bowl, mix the cornstarch and water, then add into the pan and stir, cook for 30 seconds
3. Lay the empanada wrappers on a flat surface and add the apple mixture to each one
4. Close the empanadas and roll them in half, then pinch the crust along each of the edges and roll the sides inward, continue to twist the crust until closed
5. Place the empanadas to the Air Fryer basket - It's ok to stack the empanadas inside the air fryer
6. Heat the Air Fryer on 400 degrees F and cook for 8 minutes.
7. Once done, turn and flip the empanadas, cook for an additional 10 minutes
8. Allow to cool
9. Serve!

**Nutrition Facts** Per Serving: Calories:126 |Protein: 3g |Total Fat: 1g |Total Carbs: 26g

# Lunch and Dinner

## *Cajun Shrimp with Sausage and Vegetables*

*This fast and easy Cajun Shrimp recipe is an all-in-one meal made with shrimp, sausage, and lots of colorful vegetables such as zucchini, yellow squash and bell peppers.*

Prep Time: 10 Minutes

Cook Time: 20 Minutes

Total Time: 30 Minutes

Servings: 4

## Ingredients:

- 1 tbsp Cajun or Creole seasoning
- 24 (1 lb) cleaned and peeled extra jumbo shrimp
- 6 oz fully cooked Turkey/Chicken Andouille sausage or kielbasa*, sliced
- 1 medium zucchini, 8 ounces, sliced into 1/4-inch thick half moons
- 1 medium yellow squash, 8 ounces, sliced into 1/4-inch thick half moons
- 1 large red bell pepper, seeded and cut into thin 1-inch pieces
- 1/4 tsp kosher salt
- 2 tbsp olive oil

## Directions:

1. In a large bowl, add the Cajun seasoning and shrimp, toss to coat
2. Add the sausage, squash, zucchini, bell peppers, and salt to the bowl, toss with the oil
3. Preheat the air fryer 400 F
4. In 2 batches, transfer the shrimp and vegetables to the air fryer basket and cook 8 minutes, making sure to shake the basket 2 to 3 times
5. Set aside, repeat with remaining shrimp and veggies
6. Once both batches are cooked, return the first batch to the air fryer and cook 1 minute
7. Serve hot!

**Nutrition Facts** Per Serving 1 ½: Calories:284 |Protein: 31g |Total Fat: 14g |Total Carbs: 8g

# *Zesty Herb Fish Fillets*

*Enjoy this recipe for air fried Zesty Herb Fish Fillets with a side of steamed veggies and rice!*

Prep Time: 5 Minutes

Cook Time: 12 Minutes

Total Time: 17 Minutes

Servings: 4

## Ingredients:

1. 3/4 cup bread crumbs or Panko or crush cornflakes (unsweetened)
2. 1-2 tbsp lemon herb seasoning
3. 1/2 tbsp vegetable oil
4. 2 eggs beaten
5. 4 tilapia, salmon or other fish fillets
6. Lemon wedges to garnish

## Directions:

1. Preheat your air fryer to 350 degrees F
2. In a bowl, mix the panko/breadcrumbs and the ranch dressing together, add in the oil and stir until the mixture is loose and crumbly
3. In a separate bowl, add the eggs and beat
4. Dip the fish fillets into the egg, allow the excess to drip off
5. Then dip the fish fillets into the crumb mixture, making sure to coat they are evenly coated
6. Place the fish into the air fryer
7. Air Fry for 12-13 minutes, depending on the thickness of the fillets
8. Transfer to a plate and serve with lemon wedges

**Nutrition Facts** Per Serving (Salmon): Calories:295 |Protein: 25g |Total Fat: 11g |Total Carbs: 21g

## *Lemon and Herbs Salmon Burgers*

*Skip the beef burger and opt for this delicious and quick Lemon and Herb Salmon burger! Made with fresh salmon, parsley and lemon zest, enjoy this burger with all the toppings you want.*

Prep Time: 10 Minutes

Cook Time: 10 Minutes

Total Time: 10 Minutes

Servings: 4

### Ingredients:

- 2 (6-oz) fillets of salmon, finely chopped by hand or in a food processor
- 2 eggs, lightly beaten
- 1 cup fine breadcrumbs
- 1 tsp freshly grated lemon zest
- 2 tbsp chopped fresh parsley
- 1 tbsp chopped chives
- 1 tsp salt
- freshly ground black pepper

*To Serve:*

- Brioche bun
- Avocado, sliced
- Tomato, sliced
- Lettuce, chopped
- Red onion, sliced or chopped
- Mayonnaise or Mustard

### Directions:

1. Pre-heat the air fryer to 400 degrees F
2. In a bowl, combine the chopped salmon, eggs, lemon zest, parsley, chives, breadcrumbs, salt and pepper, mix well
3. Divide the mixture into four balls, flatten the balls into patties, making an indentation in the center of each patty with your thumb and then flattening the sides of the burgers so that they fit into the air fryer basket, then transfer the burgers to the air fryer basket
4. Air fry for 5 minutes, and then flip the burgers over and air-fry for another 3 to 4 minutes, until browned and firm to the touch
5. Serve on soft brioche buns with the avocado slices, tomato, lettuce, red onion, mayo/or mustard, or the toppings of your choice

**Nutrition Facts** Per Serving: Calories:580 |Protein: 48g |Total Fat: 32g|Total Carbs: 21g

## ***Coconut Shrimp with Creamy Pineapple Dip***

*Crusted in crunchy shredded coconut and served with a creamy pineapple dip, this Coconut Shrimp recipe is a taste of the tropics you need!*

Prep Time: 15 Minutes

Cook Time: 8 Minutes

Total Time: 23 Minutes

Servings: 5

**Ingredients:**

*For the shrimp:*

- 1 1/2 lbs jumbo shrimp, devined
- 1/2 cup cornstarch
- 2/3 cup light coconut milk
- 2 tbsp honey
- 1 cup unsweetened shredded coconut
- 3/4 cup panko bread crumbs

*For the sauce:*

- 1/3 cup light coconut milk
- 1/3 cup plain nonfat Greek yogurt
- 1/4 cup pineapple chunks drained
- 1/4 tsp salt, or more to taste
- 1/4 tsp pepper, or more to taste
- Toasted coconut for garnish

**Directions:**

1. Remove the shell from the shrimp, leave the tail intact, if desired
2. Place the cornstarch in a gallon-size bag, add the shrimp, and toss to coat
3. In a medium bowl, whisk together the coconut milk and honey
4. In a separate medium bowl, combine the shredded coconut and panko
5. Remove the shrimp from bag, gently brushing off any excess cornstarch
6. Place the shrimp into the liquid mixture, then dredge in the coconut mixture, gently press any loose coconut and panko onto the shrimp
7. Transfer coated shrimp to the basket of the air fryer, working in batches since the coating comes off easily
8. Set the air fryer to 350 degrees F and cook 6 to 8 minutes, flipping shrimp once, cook until the coconut is golden brown and the shrimp is cooked thorough
9. In the meantime, prepare the sauce by combining the coconut milk, yogurt, pineapple, salt, and pepper in a bowl
10. Top with more toasted coconut
11. Enjoy with the pineapple dipping sauce!

**Nutrition Facts** Per Serving: Calories:343 |Protein: 29g |Total Fat: 12g |Total Carbs: 30g

## ***Shrimp Po Boy***

*Have a Louisiana Shrimp Po Boy with Remoulade Sauce in just 10 minutes with air fryer shrimp, fresh toppings and savory remoulade sauce.*

Prep Time: 20 Minutes

Cook Time: 10 Minutes

Total Time: 30 Minutes

Servings: 4

## Ingredients:

- 1 lb large shrimp, deveined
- 1/2 cup Louisiana fish fry or Creole fish fry
- 1/4 cup buttermilk
- 2 cups shredded lettuce
- 1 tsp creole seasoning
- 1 tsp butter, optional
- 8 tomato slices
- 1 green onion chopped
- ½ cup of Remoulade Sauce, homemade or store bought
- Olive oil cooking spray

*To Serve:*

- 4 French bread hoagie rolls I used 2 loaves, cut each in half

## Directions:

1. Season the shrimp with the creole seasoning
2. In a bowl, add the buttermilk, then dip the shrimp in the buttermilk, place the shrimp in a Ziploc bag and in the fridge to marinate for 30 minutes or overnight
3. In a bowl, add the fish fry, remove the shrimp from the bags and dip the shrimp into the fish fry
4. Place the shrimp into the Air Fryer basket
5. Preheat Air Fryer to 400 degrees F
6. Spray the shrimp with olive oil from a distance, not directly on the shrimp
7. Air fry the shrimp for 5 minutes, then open the basket and flip the shrimp to the other side, cook for an additional 5 minutes or until crisp.
8. Preheat oven to 325 degrees F and place the sliced bread on a sheet pan, allow the bread to toast for a few minutes – additionally you can melt the butter in the microwave, brush it over the bottom of the French bread and then toast
9. Assemble the Po Boy by spreading the remoulade on the bread, add the sliced tomato, lettuce and then top with the air fried shrimp
10. Enjoy!

**Nutrition Facts** Per Serving: Calories:215 |Protein: 20g |Total Fat: 6g |Total Carbs: 20g

# South of the Border Tilapia Salad

*Full of south of the border flavor, this Tortilla Crusted Tilapia Salad recipe is great as a light and healthy lunch or dinner!*

Prep Time: 15 Minutes

Cook Time: 15 Minutes

Total Time: 30 Minutes

Servings: 2

## Ingredients:

- 2 Tortilla Crusted Tilapia fillets
- 6 cup mixed greens
- 1 cup cherry tomatoes
- 1/3 cup diced red onion
- 1 avocado
- 1/2 cup Lime Ranch Dressing or Southwestern Dressing

## Directions:

1. Lightly spray the frozen tilapia fillets with cooking spray on both sides
2. Place in the Air-fryer and set the Air-fryer to 390 degrees F
3. Air-fry for 15 to 18 minutes or until crispy
4. In the meantime, in two bowls add in the half of the greens, tomatoes and red onion, toss the mixture with the lime ranch dressing
5. Top the greens with the baked fish and sliced avocado
6. Serve and enjoy!

**Nutrition Facts** Per Serving: Calories:677 |Protein: 12g |Total Fat: 45g |Total Carbs: 64g

### *Gourmet Fish Sticks*

*Forget about those freezer aisle fish sticks! Cook your own fresh and crispy gourmet fish sticks with this amazing recipe.*

Prep Time: 10 Minutes

Cook Time: 10 Minutes

Total Time: 20 Minutes

Servings: 4

## Ingredients:

- 4-6 Whiting Fish fillets cut in half
- Oil to mist
- ¾ cup very fine cornmeal
- ¼ cup flour
- Fish seasoning of your choice

## Directions:

1. In a ziplock bag, combine the fine cornmeal, flour and the fish seasoning of your choice, set aside
2. Rinse and pat dry the fish fillets with paper towels, they will still be damp
3. Place the fish fillets in ziplock bag and shake until the fillets are fully covered with seasoning
4. Then place the fillets on a baking rack to allow any excess flour fall off
5. Place the fillets in the Air Fryer basket
6. Air fry the filets on 400 degrees for 5 minutes
7. Flip and cook the other side for 5 minutes or until cooked through
8. Serve!

**Recipe Notes:** You will need to adjust the cook time depending on the thickness of the fillet

**Nutrition Facts** Per Serving: Calories:211 |Protein: 25g |Total Fat: 1g |Total Carbs: 25g

### ***Bang Bang Shrimp with Spicy Sauce***

*This Bang Bang Shrimp is awesome, quick and healthy! Plus, you can serve it up with a sweet chili and Sriracha dipping sauce.*

Prep Time: 10 Minutes

Cook Time: 20 Minutes

Total Time: 30 Minutes

Servings: 4

## Ingredients:

- 1 lb raw shrimp, peeled and deveined
- 1 egg white 3 tbsp
- 1/2 cup all-purpose flour
- 3/4 cup panko bread crumbs
- 1 tsp paprika
- Salt, to taste
- Pepper, to taste
- Chicken Seasoning, to taste
- Cooking spray

*Spicy Sauce:*

- 1/3 cup plain, non-fat Greek yogurt
- 2 tbsp Sriracha
- 1/4 cup sweet chili sauce

## Directions:

1. Preheat Air Fryer to 400 degrees F
2. Season the shrimp with the seasonings
3. In three separate bowl, divide the flour, egg whites, and panko bread crumbs
4. Create a cooking stations, dip the shrimp in the flour, then the egg whites - making sure not to submerge the shrimp, and coat with the panko bread crumbs
5. Spray the shrimp with cooking spray, don't spray directly on the shrimp, but at a distance
6. Place the shrimp to the Air Fryer basket and cook for 4 minutes, open the basket and flip the shrimp to the other side, then cook for an additional 4 minutes or until crispy
7. In a small bowl, prepare the bang bang sauce by combining the Greek yogurt, sriracha, and sweet chili sauce, stir to combine
8. Transfer the shrimp to a plate and enjoy with the bang bang sauce

**Nutrition Facts** Per Serving: Calories:242 |Protein: 37g |Total Fat: 1g |Total Carbs: 32g

# ***Spicy Mahi Mahi Tacos***

*Enjoy Taco Tuesday with this gourmet Spicy Mahi Mahi Taco recipe that is finished with all your favorite Mexican toppings!*

Prep Time: 10 Minutes

Cook Time: 9-10Minutes

Total Time: 20 Minutes

Servings: 2-3

## Ingredients:

- ½ cup flour
- 1 tsp chili powder
- ½ tsp ground cumin
- 1 tsp salt
- Freshly ground black pepper
- ½ tsp baking powder
- 1 egg, beaten
- ¼ cup milk
- 1 cup breadcrumbs
- 12 oz mahi-mahi or snapper fillets
- 1 tbsp canola or vegetable oil
- 6 (6-inch) flour tortillas
- 1 lime, cut into wedges

*Optional Toppings:*

- Avocado
- Salsa
- Jalapeno
- Cilantro
- Mexican Cabbage Slaw

## Directions:

1. In a large bowl, combine the flour, chili powder, cumin, salt, pepper and baking powder, and then add in the egg and milk, mix until the batter is smooth
2. In a shallow dish, add the breadcrumbs
3. Cut the fish fillets into 1-inch wide sticks, about 4-inches long making 12 fish sticks in total
4. Dip a fish stick into the wet batter, coating both sides - Allow the excess batter to drip off the fish
5. Then roll the fish stick in the breadcrumbs, patting the crumbs onto all sides of the fish sticks, set the coated fish on a plate or baking sheet until the remaining fish sticks are done

6. Pre-heat the air fryer to 400 degrees F
7. Place as many sticks as you can in one layer, leaving a little room around each stick, then place any remaining sticks on top, perpendicular to the first layer
8. Air-fry the fish for 5 minutes and then flip the fish sticks over and air fry for an additional 4-5 minutes.
9. In the meantime, warm the tortilla shells in the oven at 350 degrees F (wrapped in foil) or in a skillet with a little oil over medium-high heat for a few minutes - Fold the tortillas in half and keep them warm until the remaining tortillas and fish are ready
10. To assemble, place two pieces of the fish in each tortilla shell and top with toppings of your choice
11. Squeeze the lime wedge over top and enjoy!

**Nutrition Facts** Per Serving (without toppings): Calories:660 |Protein: 42g |Total Fat: 19g |Total Carbs: 77g

# ***Steak with Homemade Garlic Butter***

*Topped with homemade garlic butter, this juicy air fried steak is so amazing!*

Prep Time: 20 Minutes

Cook Time: 12 Minutes

Rest Time: 5 Minutes

Total Time: 32 Minutes

Servings: 2

## Ingredients:

- 2 (8 oz) Ribeye steak
- Salt
- Freshly cracked black pepper
- Olive oil

*Garlic Butter:*

- 1 stick unsalted butter, softened
- 2 tsp garlic, minced
- 1 tsp Worcestershire Sauce
- 2 tbsp fresh parsley, chopped
- 1/2 tsp salt

## Directions:

1. Prepare the Garlic Butter – In a bowl, mixing butter, parsley garlic, Worcestershire sauce, and salt thoroughly combined
2. Place the butter in parchment paper and roll into a log, refrigerate until ready to use
3. Remove the steak from the fridge and allow to sit at room temperature for 20 minutes
4. Rub both sided with a little bit of olive oil, then season with salt and freshly cracked black pepper
5. Preheat the Air Fryer to 400 degrees F
6. Place the steaks in the Air fryer
7. Air Fry for 12 minutes, flipping halfway through
8. Remove the steak from the Air fryer, allow to rest for 5 minutes
9. Top with garlic butter and enjoy with your favorite veggies!

**Nutrition Facts** Per Serving: Calories:568 |Protein: 48g |Total Fat: 39g |Total Carbs: 6g

# Korean-Style BBQ Beef

*Enjoy a tasty meal in 45 minutes with this Korean BBQ Beef recipe that you can serve up with rice and sautéed green beans.*

Prep Time: 15 Minutes

Cook Time: 30 Minutes

Total Time: 45 Minutes

Servings: 4

## Ingredients:

*Meat:*

- 1 lb flank steak or thinly sliced steak
- ¼ cup corn starch
- Coconut cooking spray

*Sauce:*

- 1/2 cup soy sauce
- 1/2 cup brown sugar
- 2 tbsp white wine vinegar
- 1 clove garlic, crushed
- 1 tbsp hot chili sauce
- 1 tsp ground ginger
- 1/2 tsp sesame Seeds
- 1 tbsp cornstarch
- 1 tbsp water

*To Serve:*

- Sliced green onions
- Cooked jasmine rice, or rice of your choice
- Green beans, sautéed

## Directions:

1. Prepare the steak by thinly slicing the it, and toss in the cornstarch
2. Lightly spray the steak, then place the steak in the air fryer
3. Set the Air fryer to 390 degrees F and air fry for 10 minutes, then turn the steak and cook for another 10 minutes
4. In the meantime, create the sauce by adding the soy sauce, brown sugar, white wine vinegar, garlic, hot chili sauce, ground ginger, and sesame seeds to a medium saucepan over medium heat
5. Once it reaches a low boil, then whisk in the cornstarch and water
6. Carefully remove the steak, drizzle the sauce on top, and mix well
7. Top with the sliced green onions and serve with cooked rice, and sautéed green beans

**Nutrition Facts** Per Serving: Calories:344 |Protein: 28g |Total Fat: 7g |Total Carbs: 39g

## ***Air-Fried Stuffed Peppers***

*Dig into classic ground beef roasted stuffed peppers topped with cheese in less than 30 minutes!*

Prep Time: 10 Minutes

Cook Time: 15 Minutes

Total Time: 25 Minutes

Servings: 4

## Ingredients:

- 8 oz lean ground beef
- 2 medium green peppers, stems and seeds removed, cooked in boiling salt water for 3 minutes
- ½ medium onion, chopped
- 1 clove garlic, minced
- ½ cup tomato sauce
- 1 tsp Worcestershire sauce
- 1 tsp olive oil
- ½ tsp salt
- ½ tsp black pepper
- 4 oz cheddar cheese, shredded

## Directions:

1. Preheat air fryer to 385 degrees F
2. In a pan over medium heat, sauté the onion and garlic in the olive oil until golden, allow to cool
3. In a medium bowl, combine the beef, cooked vegetables, ¼ cup tomato sauce, Worcestershire, salt and pepper and half the shredded cheese
4. Divide the mixture among the pepper halves
5. Top each one with the remaining tomato sauce and cheese
6. Arrange in the air fryer basket, work in batches if needed
7. Air fry for 15-20 minutes or until meat is cooked through
8. Enjoy!

**Nutrition Facts** Per Serving: Calories:341 |Protein: 16g |Total Fat: 27g |Total Carbs: 6g

### *Carne Asada – For Burritos, Tacos, Salads and more*

*Make everything from carne asada tacos, burritos, or a Mexican style salad with this easy Carne Asada recipe!*

Prep Time: 10 Minutes

Cook Time: 8 Minutes

Total Time: 18 Minutes

Servings: 4

## Ingredients:

- 1 ½ lbs skirt steak
- 2 medium limes, juiced
- 1 medium orange peeled and seeded
- 1 cup cilantro
- 1 jalapeno, diced
- 2 tbsp vegetable oil
- 2 tbsp vinegar
- 2 tsp ancho chile powder
- 1 tsp splenda or 2 tsp sugar
- 1 tsp salt
- 1 tsp cumin seeds
- 1 tsp coriander seeds

## Directions:

1. In blender, add the lime juice, oranges, cilantro, vegetable oil, vinegar, ancho chile, jalapeno, powder, sugar, salt, cumin and coriander seeds, mix until smooth
2. Cut the skirt steak into four pieces and place into a Ziplock bag
3. Pour in the marinade on the steak, allow the meat marinate for 30 minutes, or for 24 hours in the refrigerator
4. Preheat the Air fryer to 400 degrees F
5. Place the steaks into the air fryer basket, work in two batches if needed
6. Air fry for 8 minutes, or until the steak has reached an internal temperature of 145 degrees F, making sure to not overcook
7. Once cooked, allow the steak to rest for 10 minutes
8. Slice the steak against the grain and serve with bean and rice or in a burrito or taco

**Nutrition Facts** Per Serving: Calories:330 |Protein: 37g |Total Fat: 10g |Total Carbs: 1g

# Beef Kabobs

*Flavorful and juicy, these Beef Skewers make for an awesome meal with a side of roasted vegetables and rice.*

Prep Time: 30 Minutes

Cook Time: 10 Minutes

Total Time: 40 Minutes

Servings: 4

## Ingredients:

- 1 lb beef chuck ribs cut in 1-inch pieces or any other tender cut meat- think a nice steak, stew meat
- 1/3 cup low fat sour cream
- 2 tbsp soy sauce
- 8 (6-inch) skewers
- 1 bell peppers
- 1/2 onion

## Directions:

1. In a bowl, combine the sour cream and soy sauce
2. Add the beef chunks into the bowl and marinate for at least 30 minutes or overnight
3. Cut the bell pepper and onion in 1-inch pieces
4. In the meantime, soak the wooden skewers in water for about 10 minutes
5. Thread the beef, onions and bell peppers onto skewers, add some freshly gound black pepper
6. Cook in preheated at 400 F air fryer for 10 minutes, turning half way
7. Transfer to a plate and enjoy!

**Nutrition Facts** Per Serving: Calories:250 |Protein: 23g |Total Fat: 6g |Total Carbs: 4g

### *Marinated Steak*

*With this easy recipe you'll be able to "grill" up steaks like New York strip, ribeyes, or filet mignon in no time!*

Prep Time: 5 minutes

Cook Time: 10 minutes

Total Time: 15 minutes

Servings 2

## Ingredients:

- 2 new york strip steaks (6-8 oz each) or any cut of steak
- 1 tbsp low-sodium soy sauce
- 1 tsp liquid smoke or a cap full
- 1 tbsp steak rub
- 1/2 tbsp unsweetened cocoa powder
- Salt, to taste
- Pepper, to taste
- Melted butter, optional

## Directions:

1. Add the steak to a ziploc bag and drizzle with the soy sauce and liquid smoke
2. Then season the steak with the seasonings, refrigerate for at least a couple of hours or overnight
3. Place the steak in the air fryer, cook the two steaks at a time (if your air fryer has the space). Use a accessory grill pan, a layer rack or the standard air fryer basket
4. Cook for 5 minutes on 375 degrees F, after 5 minutes check on the steak to see if it's done with a fork or thermometer - cook to 125° F for rare, 135° F for medium-rare, 145° F for medium, 155° F for medium-well, and 160° F for well done.
5. For medium steak, at 5 minutes, flip and cooked for an additional 2 minutes, check the steaks
6. Remove the steak from the air fryer and drizzle with melted butter
7. Enjoy!

**Recipe Notes:** Trim the fat from your steak if needed.


**Nutrition Facts** Per Serving for a New York Strip: Calories:476 |Protein: 46g |Total Fat: 28g |Total Carbs: 1g

## Smoked Midwest BBQ Ribs

*Tender and juicy, you'll fall in love with these smoked BBQ ribs topped with your favorite BBQ sauce and served up with your midwest favorite sides!*

Prep Time: 35 Minutes

Cook Time: 30 Minutes

Total Time: 1 Hour 5 Minutes

Servings: 6

**Ingredients:**

- 1 rack ribs (baby back or spare ribs)
- 1/2 cup BBQ sauce, warmed
- 1 tbsp liquid smoke
- 2-3 tbsp pork rub of your choice
- Salt, to taste
- Pepper, to taste

**Directions:**

1. Remove the membrane from the back of the ribs – This is a thin layer but it can be tough to remove, you can cut it off or pull it off
2. Prepare the ribs by cutting them in half or separate all the ribs to make sure they are able to fit in the air fryer
3. Drizzle 1 tbsp of liquid smoke over both sides of the ribs
4. In a bowl combine the pork rub, salt and pepper, season both sides of the ribs
5. Cover the ribs and allow them to sit at room temperature for 30 minutes
6. Place the ribs in the air fryer - It is ok to stack the ribs
7. Set the Air fryer to 360 degrees F and cook for 15 minutes
8. Once completed, open the air fryer and flip the ribs, cook for an additional 15 minutes
9. In the meantime, warm up the BBQ sauce on the stove top
10. Remove the ribs from the air fryer
11. Drizzle the ribs with BBQ sauce
12. Enjoy!

**Nutrition Facts** Per Serving: Calories:644 |Protein: 51g |Total Fat: 47g |Total Carbs: 3g

## *Fried Garlic Chicken Wings*

*Covered in garlic and parmesan breading, these awesome Chicken Wings are crispy on the outside and juicy on the inside.*

Prep Time: 10 Minutes

Cook Time: 20 Minutes

Total Time: 30 Minutes

Servings: 4

### Ingredients:

- 16 chicken wings drummettes
- 1/4 cup low-fat buttermilk
- 1/2 cup flour
- 1/4 cup parmesan grated
- 1 tsp parmesan
- 2 tbsp low-sodium soy sauce
- 1 tsp garlic powder
- Chicken seasoning, of choice, to taste
- Pepper, to taste
- Cooking spray

### Directions:

1. Preheat the Air Fryer to 400 degrees F
2. Wash and pat dry the chicken and drizzle the soy sauce over the chicken
3. Season the chicken with the chicken seasoning, place in a Ziploc bag and marinate in the fridge for about 30 minutes or overnight
4. Once the chicken has marinated, place the flour and 1/4 cup of parmesan into a separate Ziploc bag
5. In a large bowl, pour in the buttermilk
6. Then coat the chicken with the buttermilk and add it to the Ziploc bag with the flour and parmesan, shake to thoroughly coat
7. Spray the pan with cooking oil
8. With tongs, remove the chicken from the bag and place on the Ninja Foodi Air Fryer pan - It's ok to stack the chicken on top of each other - spray with the cooking spray over the top of the chicken. Air fry for 20 minutes.
9. Allow the chicken to cook for 5 minutes - remove the pan and shake the chicken to ensure all of the pieces are fully cooked - then continue to cook and repeat shaking every 5 minutes until the 20 minutes are completed
10. Allow the chicken to cool before serving, garnish with the remaining parmesan and serve!

**Nutrition Facts** Per Serving: Calories:247 |Protein: 30g |Total Fat: 6g |Total Carbs: 15g

## *Herb Roast Chicken*

*Deliciously moist and seasoned to perfection, this herb roasted chicken is full of flavorful and crispy on the outside!*

Prep Time: 10 Minutes

Cook Time: 50 Minutes

Total Time: 60 Minutes

Servings: 4

## Ingredients:

- 4.25 lb whole chicken
- Dry rub or herb seasoning of your choice
- Cooking spray

## Directions:

1. Prepare the chicken by cleaning it, pat it dry
2. Sprinkle generously with the dry rub or the seasonings of your choice
3. Spray the fry basket with cooking spray, then place the chicken into the basket with the legs facing down.
4. Roast the chicken for 330 degrees F for 30 minutes, then flip the chicken
5. Roast for 20 more minutes at 330 degrees F or until the internal temperature reaches 165 degrees F
6. Remove from basket, slice and enjoy for lunch or dinner in a sandwich or as the main dish

### *Jerk Chicken*

*Dig into this Air Fryer Jerk Chicken that's juicy and bursting with exotic flavors!*

Prep Time: 10 Minutes

Cook Time: 10 Minutes

Total Time: 20 Minutes

Servings: 8

## Ingredients:

- 3 lbs boneless, skinless chicken thigh fillets, pat dry
- 1 tbsp ground coriander seed
- 1 tbsp ground cinnamon
- 1 tbsp cayenne pepper
- 1-1/2 tsp ground ginger
- 1-1/2 tsp ground nutmeg
- Coarse ground black pepper, to taste
- Salt, to taste
- 3 tbsp coconut oil, melted

## Directions:

1. Season the chicken thighs with salt and pepper both sides, allow the chicken sit for 30 minutes to reach room temperature
2. In a small bowl, combine the spices (coriander, cinnamon, cayenne, ginger and nutmeg), coat the chicken with the spice mixture
3. Brush both sides of the chicken with coconut oil
4. Working in batches, place four pieces of chicken into the air fryer basket – make sure they don't overlap
5. Air fry at 390 degrees F for 10 minutes or until cooked through
6. Remove the chicken from the basket, place it in an oven safe dish, and cover it tightly with foil
7. Air frying the rest of the chicken thighs
8. Serve with a fresh salad and rice

**Nutrition Facts** Per Serving: Calories:202 |Protein: 24g |Total Fat: 13g |Total Carbs: 1.7g

### *Chicken Quesadilla*

*Loaded with chicken, green pepper and gooey cheese, this easy chicken quesadilla makes for a delicious homemade lunch or quick dinner!*

Prep Time: 10 Minutes

Cook Time: 8 Minutes

Total Time: 18 Minutes

Servings: 4

**Ingredients:**

- Soft taco shells
- Chicken fajita Strips, fully cooked
- 1/2 cup sliced green peppers
- 1/2 cup thinly sliced onions, raw or sautéed
- Shredded Mexican cheese
- Salsa
- Sour cream

**Directions:**

1. Preheat the Air Fryer to 370 degrees F
2. Carefully place 1 soft taco shell in the air fryer inner basket
3. Place the shredded cheese on shell, as much you desire
4. Arrange the fajita chicken strips in a single layer, top with the onions and the green peppers
5. Then sprinkle more shredded cheese on top
6. Place another soft taco shell on top and spray lightly with vegetable oil, place the rack that comes with the air fryer on top to hold it in place
7. Air fry for 4 minutes, then flip it over carefully with a large spatula
8. Continue to air fry for 4 minutes, if it's not crispy continue to air fry for a few more minutes
9. Transfer the quesadilla to a plate and cut into 4 slices or 6 slices.
10. Serve with salsa and sour cream, if desired

**Recipe Notes:** You can also make this recipe with carne asada or steak strips!

**Nutrition Facts** Per Serving: Calories:164 |Protein: 10g |Total Fat: 10g |Total Carbs: 8g

## ***Crispy BBQ Wings***

*Fall in love with these Crispy Chicken Wings that are juicy and topped with your favorite BBQ or wing sauce!*

Prep Time: 5 Minutes

Cook Time: 30 Minutes

Total Time: 35 Minutes

Servings: 5

**Ingredients:**

- 2 lbs chicken wings cut into drumettes and flats
- 1/2 cup BBQ or wing sauce

**Directions:**

- Preheat the Air Fryer to 380 degrees F
- Pat the wings dry and place the wings in the basket and insert into the air fryer.
- Air Fry for 24 minutes, after 13 minutes, turn the wings with tongs
- Once cooked, increase the temperature to 400 degrees F and air fry for 6 more minutes or until the skin is browned and crisp
- Once completed, transfer to a bowl, add toss with your favorite BBQ or wing sauce
- Serve!

**Nutrition Facts** Per Serving: Calories:373 |Protein: 55g |Total Fat: 15g |Total Carbs: 1g

## ***Pickle-Brined Fried Chicken***

*This juicy, flavorful chicken is marinated in pickle juice, seasoned, coated with breadcrumbs and cooked to perfection!*

Prep Time: 3 hrs

Cook Time: 27 Minutes

Total Time:  3 hrs 27 Minutes

Servings: 4

### Ingredients:

- 4 chicken legs bone-in and skin-on, cut into drumsticks and thighs, about 3½ lbs
- Pickle juice from a 24-ounce jar of kosher dill pickles
- ½ cup flour
- salt and freshly ground black pepper
- 2 eggs
- 2 tbsp vegetable or canola oil
- 1 cup fine breadcrumbs
- ½ tsp ground paprika
- 1/8 tsp cayenne pepper
- 1 tsp salt
- 1 tsp freshly ground black pepper
- Vegetable or canola oil in a spray bottle

### Directions:

1. Place the chicken in a shallow dish and top with the pickle juice, cover and transfer the chicken to the refrigerator to brine in the pickle juice for 3 to 8 hours.
2. Once ready to cook, remove the chicken from the refrigerator and allow to reach room temperature. In the meantime, set up a dredging station, place the flour in a shallow dish and season well with salt and freshly ground black pepper then whisk the eggs and vegetable oil together in a second shallow dish. In a third shallow dish, combine the breadcrumbs, paprika, cayenne pepper, salt, and pepper
3. Pre-heat the air fryer to 370 degrees F
4. Remove the chicken from pickle brine, gently dry it with a clean kitchen towel then dredge each piece of chicken in the flour, dip it into the egg mixture, and then finally press it into the breadcrumb mixture to coat all sides of the chicken
5. Place the breaded chicken on a plate or baking sheet, spray all the piece with vegetable oil
6. Working in two batches, air-fry the chicken by place two chicken thighs and two drumsticks into the air fryer basket
7. Air fry for 10 minutes, then gently turn the chicken pieces over and air fry for another 10 minutes. Remove the chicken pieces and let them rest on plate, do not

cover. Finish up with the second batch of chicken, air frying for 20 minutes, turning the chicken over halfway through.
8. Then lower the temperature of the air fryer to 340 degrees F
9. Place the first batch of chicken on top of the second batch that is in the basket, air fry for an additional 7 minutes
10. Serve warm and enjoy

**Nutrition Facts** Per Serving: Calories:598 |Protein: 34g |Total Fat: 43g |Total Carbs: 17g

## *Chicken Caesar Salad*

*Topped a classic Caesar salad with air fried chicken, toss with the dressing, and finish with croutons for a healthy lunch or dinner!*

Prep Time: 10 Minutes

Cook Time: 12 Minutes

Total Time: 22 Minutes

Servings: 4

**Ingredients:**

- 2 tbsp olive oil
- 2 tbsp fresh lemon juice
- 2 tbsp Worcestershire sauce
- 2 tbsp honey
- ½ tsp dried thyme
- ½ tsp dried oregano
- 1 tsp salt
- ¼ tsp fresh ground black pepper
- 2 (6-oz) chicken breasts
- 3 hearts romaine lettuce, washed and torn into pieces
- Parmigiano-Reggiano Cheese, shaved
- Caesar Dressing
- Garlic Parmesan Croutons

**Directions:**

1. In a small bowl, combine the olive oil, lemon juice, honey, thyme, oregano, Worcestershire sauce, salt and freshly ground black pepper
2. Place the chicken breasts in a Ziplock bag and add the marinade, marinate the chicken in the refrigerator for 6 hours or overnight
3. Pre-heat the air fryer to 380 degrees F
4. Transfer the marinated chicken breasts to the air fryer basket
5. Air fry for 12 minutes, flip the chicken over halfway through the cooking process.
6. In the meantime, place the romaine lettuce in a large bowl and drizzle the Caesar dressing on top, toss to coat
7. Add on the freshly ground black pepper, some shaved Parmigiano-Reggiano cheese and the croutons Toss and divide the salad among four plates
8. Once completed, transfer the chicken breasts to a cutting board and allow them rest for a few minutes Slice the chicken breasts on the bias and spread a few slices on top of the lettuce
9. Serve and enjoy!

**Nutrition Facts** Per Serving: Calories:354 |Protein: 30g |Total Fat: 20g |Total Carbs: 11g

### ***Chicken Fried Rice***

*With just 7 ingredients, you can make this easy air fried Chicken Fried Rice as a main entree or side dish for lunch or dinner!*

Prep Time: 10 Minutes

Cook Time: 20 Minutes

Total Time: 30 Minutes

Servings: 2

## Ingredients:

- 3 cups cooked white rice, cold
- 1 cup cooked chicken, diced
- 1 cup frozen peas and carrots
- 6 tbsp soy sauce
- 1 tbsp vegetable oil
- 1/2 cup onion, diced

## Directions:

1. In a bowl, add the cold cooked white rice
2. Add in the vegetable oil and the soy sauce, mix to combine
3. Add in the frozen peas and carrots, diced onion and diced chicken and mix thoroughly
4. Pour the rice mixture into the nonstick pan or if you're using the aluminum pan then spray it with nonstick cooking spray first
5. Place the pan into the Air Fryer
6. Set the Air Fryer to 360 degrees F for 20-minutes
7. Once done, remove the pan from the Air Fryer
8. Serve and enjoy!

# *Zesty Lemon Chicken*

*Crispy with a zesty finish, serve these easy Chicken tenderloins up with your favorite side dish and veggies!*

Prep Time: 10 Minutes

Cook Time: 12 Minutes

Total Time: 22 Minutes

Servings: 6-8

## Ingredients:

- 6 chicken tenderloins breast
- 1 1/2 cups Panko crumbs
- 2 large eggs
- Kosher salt to taste
- 2 lemons halved, divided
- Extra halved lemons for additional flavor, optional

## Directions:

1. In a large bowl, beat the eggs
2. In a separate large dish, pour in the Panko
3. Prepare the chicken by coating it on both sides with the egg and then dredge both sides in the Panko crumbs
4. Place the chicken into the air fryer
5. Air fryer to 360 degrees for 12 minutes or until cooked, flipping the chicken halfway through
6. Transfer the chicken tenders to a baking pan lined with paper toweling and sprinkle with a dash of salt and squeeze over a generous amount of lemon juice with the four halves of lemon
7. Serve with extra lemon halves and enjoy!

**Nutrition Facts** Per Serving: Calories:326 |Protein: 31g |Total Fat: 14g |Total Carbs: 16g

### *Nashville Hot Chicken*

*Bring on the heat with this recipe for air fryer Nashville Hot Chicken! Enjoy it on white bread and topped with a spicy homemade hot sauce and crunchy dill pickle slices.*

Prep Time: 10 Minutes

Cook Time: 30 Minutes

Total Time: 40 Minutes

Servings: 4

**Ingredients:**

- 2 chicken breasts, cut into 6 pieces
- 2 eggs
- 1 cup buttermilk
- 2 cups all-purpose flour
- 1 tsp garlic powder
- 1 tsp onion powder
- 2 tbsp paprika
- 2 tsp salt
- 1 tsp freshly ground black pepper
- Vegetable oil

*Nashville Hot Sauce:*

- 1/4 cup butter, melted
- 3 to 4 tsp. ground red pepper
- 2 tsp dark brown sugar
- 3/4 tsp kosher salt
- 1/2 tsp smoked paprika
- 1/2 tsp garlic powder
- 1 tbsp apple cider vinegar

*To Serve:*

- 4 slices white bread
- Dill pickle slices

**Directions:**

1. Cut the chicken breasts into 2 pieces so that you have a total of 8 pieces of chicken.
2. Create a two-stage dredging station
3. In one bowl, whisk the eggs and buttermilk together
4. In a Ziplock bag, combine the flour, paprika, garlic powder, onion powder, salt and black pepper

5. Dip the chicken pieces into the egg-buttermilk mixture, then add them into the seasoned flour, coat on all sides, repeat (egg mixture and then flour mixture) one more time – make sure to coat all sides
6. Spray the chicken with vegetable oil, set aside
7. Pre-heat the air fryer to 370 degrees F and air-fry the chicken in two batches for 20 minutes, flipping the pieces over halfway through the cooking and then transfer the chicken to a plate, and repeat with the second batch of chicken
8. Lower the temperature on the air fryer to 340 degrees F, flip the chicken back over and place the first batch of chicken on top of the second batch that is in the basket
9. Air-fry the chicken for another 7 minutes
10. In the meantime, combine the cayenne pepper and salt
11. In a small sauce pan over medium heat, add the Nashville sauce ingredient (butter, ground red pepper, dark brown sugar, salt, smoked paprika, and garlic powder) whisking for 1 minute until fragrant, then remove from heat allow to cool, and add stir in the vinegar
12. Place the fried chicken on top of the white bread slices, brush the hot sauce over the chicken
13. Top with the pickle slices and enjoy!

**Nutrition Facts** Per Serving: Calories:555 |Protein: 40g |Total Fat: 18g |Total Carbs: 54g

## ***Buddha Bowl with Tofu and Red Quinoa***

*This good-for-you Buddha bowl is a yummy dish you can enjoy any day of the week! Savory and a bit sweet, it's made with heathy red quinoa, broccoli and tofu in a delicious sauce.*

Prep Time: 20 Minutes

Cook Time: 28 Minutes

Total Time: 48 Minutes

Servings: 6

**Ingredients:**

- 1 14 oz extra firm tofu
- 2 tbsp sesame oil
- 1/4 cup soy sauce
- 3 tbsp molasses or maple syrup
- 2 tbsp. lime juice
- 1 tbsp Sriracha
- 1 lb fresh romanesco or broccoli - florets only
- 3 medium carrots, peeled and thinly sliced
- 1 red bell pepper, thinly sliced
- 8 oz. fresh spinach sautéed with garlic and olive oil
- 2 cups cooked red quinoa

**Directions:**

1. Prep the tofu by wrapping the tofu in a several paper towels, set a plate on top and press out excess liquid
2. Once the excess liquid is gone and the tofu is dry, unwrap tofu and cut into very small cubes
3. In bowl, add in the sesame oil, soy sauce, molasses, lime juice, and Sriracha, whisk to combine, add in the tofu to the sauce and allow to marinate for 5--10 minutes, stirring occasionally.
4. Preheat air fryer to 370 degrees F
5. Remove the tofu from the bowl and add it into the air fryer basket – reserve the marinade for later
6. Air fry the tofu for 15 minutes, shake the basket every 5 minutes
7. In the meantime, combine the romanesco, carrots, and bell pepper in a bowl with marinade, mix well to combine
8. Once the tofu is done, remove it from the air fryer, set aside
9. Add the mixed vegetables to the air fryer basket - leave the remaining marinade in bowl
10. Cook vegetables for 5-10 minutes, shaking the basket halfway through

11. In a large serving bowl, assemble the Buddha Bowl by adding the cooked quinoa, arrange the cooked veggies evenly on top, add the cooked spinach and top with the tofu. Pour over the remaining marinade and garnish with sesame seeds
12. Enjoy!

**Nutrition Facts** Per Serving: Calories:157 |Protein: 9g |Total Fat: 6g |Total Carbs: 17g

## *Spicy Cauliflower Stir-Fry*

*Add a little heat to the menu with this spicy cauliflower stir-fry!*

Prep Time: 5 minutes

Cook Time: 25 minutes

Total Time: 30 minutes

Servings 4

### Ingredients:

- 1 head cauliflower cut into florets
- 3/4 cup onion white, thinly sliced
- 5 cloves garlic finely sliced
- 1 1/2 tbsp tamaro or gluten free tamari
- 1 tbsp rice vinegar
- 1/2 tsp coconut sugar
- 1 tbsp Sriracha or other favorite hot sauce
- 2 scallions for garnish

### Directions:

1. Place the cauliflower in the air fryer - If the air fryer has holes in the bottom, use an air fryer insert
2. Cook at 350 degrees F for 10 minutes
3. Shake the cauliflower up by opening the air fryer, grabbing the pot by the handle, remove and shake and slide back in the compartment
4. Add in the sliced onion, stir and cook for 10 more minutes
5. Add in garlic, stir and cook 5 more minutes
6. In a small bowl, mix together the soy sauce, rice vinegar, coconut sugar, Sriracha, salt and pepper
7. Pour the mixture over the cauliflower and stir, then cook for 5 more minutes.
8. To serve, garnish with sliced scallions

**Nutrition Facts** Per Serving: Calories:93 |Protein: 4g  Total Fat: 3g |Total Carbs: 12g

# ***Meatless Jackfruit Taquitos***

*You won't want to wait till Meatless Monday to enjoy these crispy and totally plant-based Jackfruit taquitos!*

Prep Time: 10 Minutes

Cook Time: 35 Minutes

Total Time: 45 Minutes

Servings: 2

## Ingredients:

- 1 14 oz can water-packed jackfruit, drained and rinsed
- 1 cup cooked or canned red beans, drained and rinsed
- 4 6-inch corn or whole wheat tortillas
- 1/2 cup pico de gallo sauce
- 1/4 cup plus 2 tbsp water
- 4 spritzes canola oil or extra-virgin olive oil

## Directions:

1. In a medium saucepan over medium heat, combine the jackfruit, beans, pico de gallo, and water bring to a boil, then reduce the heat, cover the saucepan, and simmer for 20 to 25 minutes
2. With or fork or masher, mash the jackfruit mixture into a shredded meaty texture
3. Preheat the air fryer to 370 degrees F for 3 minutes
4. Place a tortilla on a work surface, spoon 1/4 cup of the jackfruit mixture onto the tortilla
5. Roll it up tightly, pushing any of the mixture that may fall out back into the tortilla
6. Repeat and create 4 taquitos
7. Spritz the tops of the tortillas with cooking spray
8. Place the rolled tortillas into the air fryer basket, air fry at 370 degrees F for 8 minutes
9. Enjoy with salsa

**Nutrition Facts** Per Serving: Calories:574 |Protein: 19g |Total Fat: 9g |Total Carbs: 109g

### ***Stir Fried Zoodles with Vegetables and Tofu***

*Whip up delicious Asian stir fry with zoodles, vegetables and firm tofu covered in a sweet and savory sauce in your air fryer.*

Prep time:  20 minutes

Cook time:  30 minutes

Total time:  50 minutes

Serves: 4

## Ingredients:

- 1 tbsp canola oil
- 1 lbs extra firm tofu, cubed
- ½ onion, sliced
- 2 carrots, sliced
- 1 red bell pepper, sliced
- 1 cup snow peas, sliced lengthwise
- 1 can baby corn, drained
- 8 oz spiralized zucchini, zoodles
- 2 tbsp rice wine vinegar
- 2 tbsp brown rice syrup or honey
- 2 tbsp sriracha chili sauce
- 2 tbsp soy sauce
- 1 tbsp sesame oil
- 1 tsp minced fresh ginger
- Fresh cilantro leaves

## Directions:

1. In a bowl, combine the canola oil, brown rice syrup, sriracha chili sauce, rice wine vinegar, soy sauce, sesame oil, and ginger
2. Add the tofu and allow marinate for 15 minutes
3. Pre-heat the air fryer to 400 degrees F
4. Remove the tofu from the marinade with a slotted spoon and transfer it to the air fryer basket, reserve the marinade for later
5. Air-fry the tofu for 15 minutes, until the tofu is brown and crispy, shaking the basket a few times while the tofu cooks
6. Remove from the air fryer, set it aside

7.  Add the onion and carrots to the air fryer, air-fry at 400 degrees F for 5 minutes, then add in the red pepper, snow peas and baby corn, air-fry for another 5 minutes, then toss in the zucchini, air-fry for another 5 minutes, shaking the basket once during the cooking process.
8.  Add the tofu back into the air fryer basket with the vegetables and pour in the reserved marinade, toss to coat
9.  Air-fry for a few minutes, or until the vegetables are tender and heated
10. Once done, transfer to a plate with the sauce, top with the fresh cilantro

**Nutrition Facts** Per Serving: Calories:322 |Protein: 16g |Total Fat: 14g |Total Carbs: 39g

## *Crispy Eggplant Parmesan*

*Topped with marinara sauce and fresh mozzarella cheese, this crusted Eggplant parmesan makes for an awesome dinner or lunch with a side of pasta.*

Prep Time 15 minutes

Cook Time 25 minutes

Total Time 40 minutes

Serves:

### Ingredients:

- 1 large eggplant, around 1.25 lb
- 1/2 cup whole wheat bread crumbs
- 3 tbsp finely grated parmesan cheese
- 3 tbsp whole wheat flour
- olive oil spray
- Salt, to taste
- 1 tsp Italian seasoning mix
- 1 egg and 1 tbsp water
- 1 cup marinara sauce
- 1/4 cup grated mozzarella cheese
- Fresh parsley or basil to garnish

### Directions:

1. Prepare the eggplant by cutting eggplant into roughly 1/2" slices. Rub with some salt on both sides of the slices and leave it for at least 10-15 minutes
2. In the meantime, in a bowl mix together the egg, water and flour
3. In a medium shallow plate, combine the bread crumbs, parmesan cheese, Italian seasoning blend, and salt, mix well
4. Drench the eggplant slices in the batter evenly, dip the battered slices in the breadcrumb, mix to coat it evenly on all sides.
5. Place breaded eggplant slices on a clean and dry flat plate and spray oil on them from a distance, then spray the wire mesh of the air fryer
6. Preheat the Air Fryer to 360 degrees F
7. Place the eggplant slices on the wire mesh and cook for about 8 minutes
8. Top the air fried slices with about 1 tbsp of marinara sauce and lightly spread fresh mozzarella cheese on it
9. Cook the eggplant for another 1-2 minutes or until the cheese melts
10. Serve with your favorite pasta dish or enjoy alone!

**Nutrition Facts** Per Serving: Calories:221 |Protein: 12g |Total Fat: 5g |Total Carbs: 35g

# Appetizers and Snacks

## *Cheesy Mozzarella Cheese Sticks*

*This recipe for classic mozzarella sticks has less oil, more Italian flavors and the gooey cheese you love!*

Prep Time: 10 Minutes

Cook Time: 16 Minutes

Total Time: 26 Minutes

Servings: 5

## Ingredients:

- 10 pieces mozzarella string cheese
- 1 cup Italian breadcrumbs
- 1 egg
- 1/2 cup flour
- Salt, to taste
- Pepper, to taste

*To Serve:*

- 1 cup marinara sauce

## Directions:

1. Preheat the Air Fryer to 400 degrees F
2. In a bowl, season the Italian breadcrumbs with salt and pepper
3. In two separate bowls, add in the flour and eggs
4. One by one, dip the strings of cheese in flour, then egg and then coat with the breadcrumbs
5. Freeze the sticks for one hour to harden to maintain their shape
6. Spray the Air Fryer with the spray cooking oil for your choice
7. Add in the stick into the Air Fryer
8. Air Fry for 8 minutes and then remove the basket and flip all the stick with tongs, making sure not to change the shape of the mozzarella sticks
9. Place back inside the Air Fryer and cook for an additional 5-8 minutes
10. Allow the sticks to cool for 5 minutes, then transfer them to a plate – If cheese leaks from the sticks, allow them to completely cool and then use your hands to correct the shape.
11. Serve!

**Nutrition Facts** Per Serving: Calories:199 |Protein: 15g |Total Fat: 2g |Total Carbs: 30g

## *Crispy Avocado Fries with Lime Dipping Sauce*

*Coated with panko breadcrumbs, these Avocado fries are crispy, golden and perfect for dipping!*

Prep Time: 7 Minutes

Cook Time: 8 Minutes

Total Time: 15 Minutes

Servings: 6

### Ingredients:

- 8 oz. (2 small) avocados, peeled, pitted and cut into 16 wedges
- 1 large egg, lightly beaten
- 3/4 cup panko breadcrumbs
- 1 1/4 tsp lime chili seasoning salt

*For the lime dipping sauce:*

- 1/4 cup 0% Greek Yogurt
- 3 tbsp light mayonnaise
- 2 tsp fresh lime juice
- 1/2 tsp lime chili seasoning salt
- 1/8 tsp kosher salt

### Directions:

- Preheat the Air Fryer to 390 degrees F
- In a shallow bowl, add the eggs and lightly beat
- In a sperate bowl, combine the panko with 1 tsp Tajin
- Season avocado wedges with 1/4 tsp Tajin, dip each avocado wedge in egg, and then coat with the panko
- Spray both sides with the oil and then transfer the wedges to the air fryer
- Air Fry for 7 to 8 minutes, turn them halfway through
- Serve the avocado fries hot with the lime dipping sauce or a dipping sauce of your choice
- Enjoy!

**Nutrition Facts** Per Serving: Calories:104 |Protein: 1g |Total Fat: 9g |Total Carbs: 4g

# Sweet and Spicy Honey Chicken Wings

*These delicious Sweet and Spicy Chicken Wings are made with zero oil and an amazing crowd pleaser!*

Prep Time: 10 Minutes

Cook Time: 30 Minutes

Total Time: 40 Minutes

Servings: 6

## Ingredients:

- 1 lbs chicken wings, tips removed and wings cut into individual drummettes and flats.
- 1/4 cup honey
- 2 tbsp sriracha sauce
- 1 1/2 tbsp soy sauce
- 1 tbsp butter
- Juice of 1/2 lime

*Garnish:*

- Cilantro, chives, or scallions

## Directions:

1. Preheat the air fryer to 360 degrees F
2. Add the chicken wings to the air fryer basket, and cook for 30 minutes - turn the chicken every 7 minutes with tongs to evenly brown the chicken
3. In the meantime, add the sriracha sauce, soy sauce, honey, butter and lemon juice into a small sauce pan and bring it a boil for about 3 minutes
4. Once the wings are cooked, toss them in a bowl with the sauce and fully coated them
5. Sprinkle with the garnish, and enjoy!

**Nutrition Facts** Per Serving: Calories:161 |Protein: 17g |Total Fat: 5g |Total Carbs: 13g

## *Crispy Onion Rings*

*With just 6-Ingredient, these onion rings are surprisingly crispy, and golden brown! Plus, you won't get splattered with oil as you cook them.*

Prep Time: 10 Minutes

Cook Time: 30 Minutes

Total Time: 40 Minutes

Servings: 6

**Ingredients:**

- 2-3 yellow onions (3 medium or 2 large), peeled

*For the wet mix:*

- 1/2 cup flour of choice
- 2/3 cup unsweetened milk, of choice
- 1/2 tsp paprika
- 1/4 tsp turmeric
- 1/2 tsp salt

*For the dry mix:*

- 1 cup panko bread crumbs
- 1/2 tsp paprika
- 1/4 tsp turmeric
- 1/4 tsp salt

**Directions:**

1. Preheat the Air Fryer to 400 degrees F
2. Slice the end off of each onion, and peel off the outer skin, then carefully cut each onion into 1/2" circular portions. Using your fingers, carefully press the center portion of onion away from two of the onion layers to form a hollow ring. Repeat this step until no more circles remains and continue with the rest of the onion portions.
3. In a medium bowl, combine the wet mix (the flour, unsweetened milk, paprika, turmeric and salt)
4. In a separate medium bowl, combine the dry mix (panko bread crumbs paprika, turmeric and salt)
5. Then, divide the dry Mix evenly into two separate bowls to prevent the mixture from becoming sticky
6. Prepare the onion rings by using separate hands for the Wet and Dry mixes, dip the Onion Ring into the Wet Mix, then transfer it to the Dry Mix and coat with breadcrumbs
7. Place the onion rings into the Air Fryer Basket

8. Air Fry for 8-10 minutes – cook in batches and make sure the basket isn't overcrowded
9. Transfer the onion rings to a plate
10. Once done, allow the onion rings to cool
11. Serve warm and enjoy!

**Nutrition Facts** Per Serving: Calories:87 |Protein: 3g |Total Fat: 1g |Total Carbs: 17g

## *Bacon Wrapped Jalapeño Poppers*

*You can't go wrong with these easy bacon and cream cheese stuffed jalapeño poppers!
They make for a great snack or appetizer.*

Prep Time: 10 Minutes

Cook Time: 5 Minutes

Total Time: 15 Minutes

Servings: 5

### Ingredients:

- 10 fresh jalapenos, sliced in half
- 6 oz. cream cheese or reduced-fat
- 1/4 cup shredded cheddar cheese
- 2 slices bacon, cooked and crumbled
- cooking oil spray
- Salt, to taste, if desired
- Pepper, to taste, if desired

*Needed:*

- Gloves, for cutting the jalapeños

### Directions:

1. Preheat the Air fryer to 370 degrees F
2. Slice the jalapeños in half, vertically and remove the seeds inside the jalapenos (if you like things spicy, keep some seeds), set aside
3. In a bowl, add the cream cheese and microwave for 15 seconds or until to soften
4. In the same bowl, combine the cream cheese, crumbled bacon, and shredded, mix well to combine - For extra spicy poppers, add some of the seeds you set aside into the cream cheese mixture and mix well
5. Stuff the cream cheese mixture into each of the jalapeños
6. Place the poppers into the Air Fryer and spray cooking oil spray
7. Air Fry for 5 to 8 minutes or until brown and the popper are to your preference (soft or crunchy)
8. Once done, remove the poppers from the Air Fryer and allow to cool
9. Serve!

**Recipe Notes:** Salt isn't added to this recipe because of the bacon, but feel free to add salt and pepper if needed.

**Nutrition Facts** Per Serving: Calories:198 |Protein: 6g |Total Fat: 13g |Total Carbs: 15g

# ***Sugared Dippers with Chocolate Sauce***

*Satisfy your sweet tooth with this recipe for sugar dough dippers paired with a creamy chocolate Amaretto Sauce!*

Prep Time: 10 Minutes

Cook Time: 25 Minutes

Total Time: 35 Minutes

Servings: 8

## Ingredients:

- 1 lb bread dough, defrosted
- ½ cup butter, melted
- 12 oz semi-sweet chocolate chips, good quality
- 2 tbsp Amaretto liqueur (or almond extract)
- 1 cup heavy cream
- ¾ to 1 cup sugar

## Directions:

1. Prepare the dough by rolling it into two 15-inch logs, cut each log into 20 slices, then cut each slice in half and twist the dough into halves together 3 to 4 times
2. Place the twisted dough on a cookie sheet, brush with the melted butter and sprinkle sugar over the dough twists
3. Prepare the air fryer by brushing the bottom of it with melted butter
4. Pre-heat the air fryer to 350 degrees F
5. Working in batches, place 8 to 12 twists into the air fryer basket
6. Air-fry for 5 minutes, turn the dough strips over and brush the other side with butter and continue to air-fry for an additional 3 minutes
7. In the meantime, make the chocolate amaretto sauce by bring the heavy cream to a simmer over medium heat. In a large bowl, add the chocolate chips and pour the hot cream over the chocolate chips, stir with a wire whisk until the chocolate starts to melt. Whisk until the chocolate is completely melted and the sauce is smooth. Stir in the Amaretto liqueur and then pour the sauce into a serving dish
8. Once the dough twists are done, place them into a shallow dish, brush them with melted butter and generously coat with sugar, shaking the dish to cover both sides
9. Enjoy the warm sugared dough dippers with the warm chocolate Amaretto sauce

**Nutrition Facts** Per Serving: Calories:586 |Protein: 7g |Total Fat: 30g |Total Carbs: 63g

# Garlic Fried Chicken Wings

*Enjoy the bold garlic taste of these Air Fried Garlic Fried Chicken Wings in just 20 minutes!*

Prep Time: 10 Minutes

Cook Time: 20 Minutes

Total Time: 30 Minutes

Servings: 4

## Ingredients:

- 16 chicken wings drummettes
- 1/4 cup low-fat buttermilk
- 1/2 cup flour
- 1/4 cup parmesan grated
- 1 tsp parmesan
- 2 tbsp low-sodium soy sauce
- 1 tsp garlic powder
- Chicken seasoning, of choice, to taste
- Pepper, to taste
- cooking spray

## Directions:

1. Preheat the Air Fryer to 400 degrees F
2. Wash and pat the dry chicken
3. Drizzle the soy sauce over the chicken, season the chicken with the chicken seasoning, place in a Ziploc bag and marinate in the fridge for about 30 minutes or overnight
4. Once the chicken has marinated, place the flour and 1/4 cup of parmesan into a separate Ziploc bag
5. In a large bowl, pour in the buttermilk, then coat the chicken with the buttermilk and add it to the Ziploc bag with the flour and parmesan, shake to thoroughly coat
6. Spray the pan with cooking oil
7. With tongs, remove the chicken from the bag and place on the Air fryer pan – stacking is ok - spray with the cooking spray over the top of the chicken
8. Air fry for 20 minutes, then allow the chicken to cook for 5 minutes - remove the pan and shake the chicken to ensure all of the pieces are fully cooked. Continue to cook and repeat shaking every 5 minutes until the 20 minutes are completed
9. Allow the chicken to cool before serving
10. Garnish with the remaining parmesan and enjoy!

**Nutrition Facts** Per Serving: Calories:247 |Protein: 30g |Total Fat: 6g |Total Carbs: 15g

### *Crispy Chickpeas*

*Have a healthy, tasty and crunchy snack in 20 minutes with this recipe for crispy air fryer chickpeas!*

Prep Time: 5 Minutes

Cook Time: 15 Minutes

Total Time: 20 Minutes

Servings: 4

**Ingredients:**

- 19 oz can of chickpeas, drained and rinsed
- 1 tbsp olive oil
- 1/8 tsp salt
- 1/4 tsp garlic powder
- 1/4 tsp onion powder
- 1/2 tsp paprika
- 1/4 tsp cayenne, optional

**Directions:**

1. Preheat the air fryer to 390 degrees F
2. Drain and rinse the can of chickpeas, toss with olive oil and spices (garlic, salt, onion powder, paprika, and cayenne)
3. Place the chickpeas in the air fryer basket
4. Air fry for 12to 15 minutes or until the chickpeas are cooked and browned to your liking, shaking a few times while cooking
5. Remove the chickpeas from the air fryer, taste and season with more salt and pepper, if desired
6. Enjoy!

**Recipe Notes:** If you'd like to up the flavors you could try tossing in a spice blends of your choice

**Nutrition Facts** Per Serving ¼ batch: Calories:251 |Protein: 11g |Total Fat: 6g |Total Carbs: 36g

## *Citrus Lime Shrimp Skewers*

*These Citrus Lime Air Fryer Shrimp Skewers make for perfect party appetizers and tasty snacks!*

Prep Time: 5 Minutes

Cook Time: 8 Minutes

Total Time: 13 Minutes

Servings: 4

### Ingredients:

- 1/2 lb raw shrimp, peeled and deveined
- 1/2 tsp garlic purée
- 1/2 tsp paprika
- 1/2 tsp ground cumin
- Juice of 1 lime
- 1/2 of an orange, juiced
- Salt, to taste
- 1 tbsp of chopped cilantro or fresh coriander leaves

### Directions:

1. Prepare the 6 wooden skewers by soaking them for 15-20 mins before needed
2. Preheat air fryer to 350 degrees F
3. In a bowl, combine the lemon juice, garlic, paprika, cumin and salt
4. Add in the shrimp, stir to evenly coat
5. Thread the shrimp onto the skewers
6. Place the skewers into the air fryer - make sure they are not touching
7. Air fry for 5-8 mins or until done, turning skewers halfway through the cook time.
8. Transfer shrimp to a plate
9. Serve with chopped cilantro (coriander) and extra lime slices!

**Nutrition Facts** Per Serving: Calories:59 |Protein: 11g |Total Fat: 0g |Total Carbs: 1g

## *Spiced Sweet Potato Fries*

*Sweet, savory and crispy, make a healthy batch of crispy sweet potato fries with just a small amount of oil!*

Prep Time: 5 Minutes

Cook Time: 5 Minutes

Total Time: 10 Minutes

Servings: 3

### Ingredients:

- 2 medium peeled sweet potatoes (12 oz total)
- 2 tsp olive oil
- 1/2 tsp garlic powder
- 1/4 tsp sweet paprika
- 1/2 tsp kosher salt
- Fresh black pepper, to taste
- Olive oil cooking spray

### Directions:

1. Preheat air fryer to 400 degrees F
2. Lightly spray the fryer basket with the olive oil cooking spray
3. Slice each one of the sweet potatoes into even 1/4-inch-thick fries
4. In a bowl, toss the sweet potatoes with the oil, garlic powder, salt, black pepper and paprika
5. While working in batches and making sure not to overcrowd the air fryer, cook for 8 minutes, turn half way and continue to cook for 6 minutes or until done
6. Enjoy as a snack or with guests

**Recipe Note:** Add more sweet potatoes if you planning to serve these as an appetizer

**Nutrition Facts** Per Serving (1 sweet potato): Calories:221 |Protein: 3g |Total Fat: 5g |Total Carbs: 42g

# *Fried Italian Ravioli*

*Ravioli doesn't always need to be the main dish; this time treat yourself to crispy fried ravioli and served up with marinara sauce and a sprinkle of cheese as an appetizer or snack.*

Prep Time: 15 Minutes

Cook Time: 9 Minutes

Total Time: 24 Minutes

Servings: 5

## Ingredients:

- 1 (10 oz) package of refrigerated ravioli, brand of your choice
- 1 cup Italian style Bread Crumbs
- 3/4 cup Parmesan cheese, divided shredded, and roughly chop
- 3 eggs, beaten
- 1/2 tsp garlic salt
- Marinara sauce, to serve
- Fresh parsley, to serve

## Directions:

1. Preheat the Air Fryer to 350 degrees F
2. Microwave a medium sized bowl of water until boiling
3. Add in the ravioli for about 5 minutes, then drain
4. In a bowl, combine the bread crumbs with 1/2 cup or Parmesan cheese
5. In a separate bowl, beat the eggs with the garlic salt
6. In another bowl, add the seasoned bread crumbs
7. Line the bowls up and dip the ravioli in egg then press it into the bread crumbs - making sure to coat evenly on both sides
8. Fill the basket of the air fryer with a single layer of ravioli
9. Air fry for 9 minutes, then remove the ravioli and transfer to a plate
10. Serve with marinara, fresh parsley and shredded Parmesan cheese

**Nutrition Facts** Per Serving: Calories:223 |Protein: 12g |Total Fat: 12g |Total Carbs: 15g

## *Cinnamon Apple Chips*

*Satisfy your sweet tooth in the healthiest way with this recipe for crisp, delicious cinnamon apple chips!*

Prep Time: 5 Minutes

Cook Time: 8 Minutes

Total Time: 13 Minutes

Yields: 3 cups

**Ingredients:**

- 3 large sweet, crisp apples
- 3/4 tsp ground cinnamon or apple pie spice blend
- A pinch of salt

**Directions:**

1. Wash the apples thoroughly in warm water or with apple cider vinegar, rinse. Then core the apples or leave the seeds in, if preferred
2. Preheat the air fryer at 390 degrees F.
3. Using a mandolin or sharp knife, cut the apple sideways into 1/8th inch rounds.
4. In a bowl, combine the cinnamon and salt
5. Arrange the apples in a single layer on a flat surface. Sprinkle and rub with some of the cinnamon and salt mixture
6. Working in batches, arrange a single layer of the apple slices in the air fryer
7. Air fry for 8 minutes, flipping sides half way through
8. Once completed, allow the chips to cool on a cooling rack
9. Enjoy right away or store them into an air tight container for later

**Nutrition Facts** Per Serving (1 cup): Calories:65 |Protein: 0g |Total Fat: 0g |Total Carbs: 18g

### ***Crispy Plantains***

*Simple to make and ready in just 10 minutes, you'll love having these air fryer Plantains as a snack!*

Prep Time: 2 Minutes

Cook Time: 8 Minutes

Total Time: 10 Minutes

Servings: 2

## Ingredients:

- 1 plantain
- 3/4 tsp oil
- Salt to taste

*Spices:*

- Cinnamon
- Cardamom
- Nutmeg

## Directions:

- Preheat air fryer to 350 degrees F
- Peel the plantain, cut it into slices and add the slices into a bowl
- Gently mix in the oil and salt until plantains are thoroughly coated on both sides
- Arrange half of the plantain slices in the air fryer basket in a single layer, making sure that the plantains don't touch each other
- Cook for 10 minutes or until crisp, turning half way through
- Serve warm

**Nutrition Facts** Per Serving - Calories: 124| Protein: 1g | Total Fat: 2g| Total Carbs: 28g

# Banana & PB Wonton Bites

Prep Time: 15 Minutes

*Air Fryer Banana and PB Wonton Bites are easy to make and can be enjoyed alone or with a side of vanilla ice cream!*

Cook Time: 6 Minutes

Total Time: 21 Minutes

Servings: 4

## Ingredients:

- 1 large banana, sliced
- 12 won ton wrappers
- 1/2 cup peanut butter
- 1-2 tsp vegetable oil, or coconut, avocado oil
- 1 oil mister

*Add-Ins:*

- Chocolate Chips, raisins, M&M's, or ground cinnamon

## Directions:

1. Place the slice banana in a small bowl of water with a splash of lemon to prevent them from browning
2. Assemble the wontons by placing one banana slice, and 1 tsp of peanut butter and an add-in of your choice in the middle of wrapper
3. Brush along the edges of the wrapper with water. Bring together the opposite corners and squeeze, then fold up the remaining opposite sides and squeeze
4. Spray the wontons with oil, then place the prepared wonton wrappers into the air fryer
5. Air fry at 380 degrees F for 6 minutes or until golden brown
6. Serve with a scoop of vanilla ice cream and a dash of cinnamon and sugar

**Nutrition Facts** Per Serving - Calories:278| Protein: 8g | Total Fat: 6g| Total Carbs: 47g

### *Sweet Banana & Nutella Sandwich*

*Decadent hazelnut + ripe bananas, you can't go wrong with this naturally sweet and perfectly toasted sandwich!*

Prep Time: 10 Minutes

Cook Time: 8 Minutes

Total Time: 18 Minutes

Servings: 2

## Ingredients:

- Butter, softened
- 4 slices white bread
- ¼ cup chocolate hazelnut spread
- 1 banana

## Directions:

1. Pre-heat the air fryer to 370 degrees F
2. Using a butter knife, gently spread the softened butter on one side of each bread slice, then place the slices, buttered side down on a baking tray
3. With a different butter knife, spread the chocolate hazelnut spread on the other side of the bread slices. Prepare the banana by slicing it in half and then slice each half into three slices lengthwise, then place the banana slices on only two slices of bread
4. Top the banana slices with the remaining slices of bread to create two sandwiches
5. Cut the sandwiches in half – to fit them all into the air fryer at once - then transfer the sandwiches to the air fryer.
6. Air-fry for 5 minutes
7. Once done, flip the sandwiches over and air-fry for another 2-3 minutes, or until the top bread slices have browned
8. Enjoy with a glass of milk

**Nutrition Facts** Per Serving - Calories:509 | Protein: 10g | Total Fat: 20g| Total Carbs: 73g

## ***Easy Gooey Chocolate Cake***

*Bake a delicious homemade chocolate cake without touching your oven with this easy air fryer recipe!*

Prep Time: 10 Minutes

Cook Time: 25 Minutes

Total Time: 35 Minutes

Servings: 4

## **Ingredients:**

- 3 eggs
- 1/2 cup sour cream
- 1 cup flour
- 2/3 cup sugar
- 1 stick butter room temperature
- 1/3 cup cocoa powder
- 1 tsp baking powder
- 1/2 tsp baking soda
- 2 tsp vanilla

*Topping:*

- Chocolate icing

## **Directions:**

1. Preheat Air fryer to 320 degrees F
2. In a bowl, combine the eggs, sour cream, flour, sugar, butter, cocoa powder, baking powder, baking soda and vanilla with a mixer on low
3. Pour the batter into oven attachment
4. Place in Air fryer basket and air fry for 25 minutes
5. Once done, check the center of the cake with a toothpick to see if the cake is done, if not cook for an additional 5 minutes
6. Allow the cake to cool on a wire rack
7. Top with your favorite chocolate icing and enjoy!

**Nutrition Facts** Entire Cake - Calories:573 | Protein: 41g | Total Fat: 134g| Total Carbs: 253g

## Classic S'mores

*Who said you need a campfire to make s'more?! Just stack Graham crackers, marshmallow and chocolate, and cook it perfectly in your airfryer to bring back childhood memories!*

Prep Time: 5 Minutes

Cook Time: 5 Minutes

Total Time: 10 Minutes

Servings: 2

**Ingredients:**

- 2 graham crackers, in half
- 2 marshmallows, in half
- 2 small pieces of chocolate

**Directions:**

1. Place the Graham cracker halves into the bottom of Air fryer
2. The place the sticky side of broken marshmallow on top of the Graham Cracker, pushing down a little bit to sticks to the cracker.
3. Air Fry at 390 degrees F for 5-7 minutes, or until the top of the marshmallows is golden color
4. Once done, add the piece of chocolate on top of the marshmallows with the other half of the graham cracker
5. Enjoy!

**Nutrition Facts** Per Serving: Calories:249 | Protein: 3g | Total Fat: 13g| Total Carbs: 29g

## *Buffalo Cauliflower Bites*

*Vegan, and gluten-free, these delicious and healthy buffalo cauliflower bites are so amazing!*

Prep Time: 5 Minutes

Cook Time: 15 Minutes

Total Time: 20 Minutes

Servings: 4

**Ingredients:**

- 1 head cauliflower, cut into small bite
- 1/2 cup buffalo sauce
- 1 tbsp butter, melted
- Salt, to taste
- Pepper, to taste
- Cooking oil spray

*Garnish:*

- Cilantro

**Directions:**

1. Preheat the Air Fryer to 400 degrees F
2. Spray the Air Fryer basket with the cooking oil
3. In a bowl, add in the melted butter, buffalo sauce, and salt and pepper, stir to combine and set aside
4. Add the cauliflower bites to the air fryer, spray with cooking oil
5. Air Fry for 7 minutes
6. Once completed, transfer the cauliflower to a large mixing bowl, drizzle with the butter and buffalo mixture throughout, stir to coat
7. Place the cauliflower back into the air fryer
8. Set the Air Fryer to 400 degrees F and cook for an additional 5 to 8 minutes or until the cauliflower wings are crisp
9. Once cooked, transfer the cauliflower to a plate
10. Serve with Ranch Dressing or more spicy Buffalo sauce

**Nutrition Facts** Per Serving: Calories:59 |Protein: 2g |Total Fat: 3g |Total Carbs: 6g

# *Parmesan Zucchini Tater Tots*

*Way healthier than your average tater tots, these tots are full of Italian flavors and are perfect for snacking and dipping!*

Prep Time: 10 Minutes

Cook Time: 20 Minutes

Total Time: 30 Minutes

Servings: 4

## Ingredients:

- 1 large egg
- 1 1/2 cups shredded and lightly patted dry zucchini (1 1/2 medium zucchini)
- 1 cup panko bread crumbs
- 1/2 tbsp dry Italian seasoning
- 1/2 cup shredded parmesan cheese

*Dipping:*

- Ranch dressing
- Buffalo Sauce

## Directions:

1. With a vegetable grater, shred zucchini, then pat the zucchini dry with a few sheets of paper towels – it doesn't need to be totally dry, just absorb the excess moisture
2. Preheat the air fryer to 375 degrees F
3. In a large mixing bowl, measure out 1 1/2 cups of patted dry zucchini, then add in the egg, cheese and breadcrumbs, stir well to combine
4. With a spoon, take 1 tbsp of zucchini batter and squeeze between palm of hand, compressing it – while you do this some of the water will also release out
5. Then use both of your hands to shape the mixture into a cylinder tater tot shape
6. Carefully place the tater tots into the air fryer
7. Air fry for 15-20 minutes until the bottoms are golden brown and crispy, flip and bake for another 5 minutes
8. Repeat with remaining zucchini tots
9. Serve warm with the dipping sauce of your choice

**Nutrition Facts** Per Serving: Calories:188 |Protein: 9g |Total Fat: 6g |Total Carbs: 23g

### ***Spiced Bacon Wrapped Chicken***

*Spiced with a sweet and spicy rub, these Air Fried Bacon Wrapped Chicken will please all your party guests!*

Prep Time: 10 Minutes

Cook Time: 13 Minutes

Total Time: 23 Minutes

Servings: 4

## Ingredients:

- 1 lb chicken breast, cut into 1-inch pieces
- 6 slices bacon cut into thirds*
- 1/3 cup brown sugar
- 1/2 tbsp chili powder
- 1/8 tsp cayenne pepper

## Directions:

1. Place a 1-inch piece of chicken the end of a piece of bacon
2. Roll it up and secure the chicken pieces with a toothpick
3. In a bowl, combine the brown sugar, chili powder, and cayenne pepper, stir to mix
4. Coat each of the bacon wrapped chicken with the mixture, set aside
5. Place bacon wrapped chicken pieces into Air Fryer Basket - making sure there is space in between them Air fry at 390 Degrees F for 13-15 minutes
6. Once done, transfer to a plate and serve!

**Nutrition Facts** Per Serving: Calories:339 |Protein: 28g |Total Fat: 16g |Total Carbs: 18g

# Conclusion

You've now reached the end of my Best Collection of Air Fryer Recipes For Your Home cookbook! I hope you enjoy creating and sharing these easy meals with family and friends. As always, feel free to get creative and add your own twist to these recipes!

9 781693 531231